Procedures in vascular surgery

Procedures in vascular surgery

SECOND EDITION

Chilton Crane, M.D.

Clinical Professor of Surgery, Harvard Medical School; Surgeon, Peter Bent Brigham Hospital, Boston; Chief of Vascular Surgery, West Roxbury Veterans Administration Hospital, West Roxbury, Massachusetts

Richard Warren, M.D.

Professor of Surgery Emeritus, Harvard Medical School; Surgeon Emeritus, Peter Bent Brigham Hospital, Boston

ILLUSTRATED BY HARRIET R. GREENFIELD

LITTLE, BROWN AND COMPANY, BOSTON

Preface

The first edition of *Procedures in Vascular Surgery* by one of us (R. W.) appeared fifteen years ago. It was one of the first books to bring together a clear description of the core operations of a fast-growing new field—vascular surgery.

Many facets of this field of surgery remain unchanged. The indications for operation are primarily based on established criteria for clinical need, with such laboratory aids as lung scans, renal vein renin values, or pulse/volume recordings as backup support. Precise angiographic delineation of the vascular disease continues to dictate the plan of operation. Early control of vessel inflow and outflow stands as the first rule of operation. Careful dissection just outside the adventitia and meticulous tight suturing are basic steps to success. The prohibitive cost of bleeding and infection after vascular reconstruction calls for perfection in hemostasis and asepsis. Perhaps only in neurologic, orthopedic, and cardiac surgery are faults in operative strategy and tactics so quickly brought home to both surgeon and patient.

During these fifteen years, major advances in allied disciplines have extended the useful application of these basic principles. Improved instrumentation, better knowledge of flows and gradients, and newer approaches to old operations have broadened the field and improved results. Some, like the Fogarty catheter and perhaps the Sparks mandril, derived from innovative bioengineering, have been breakthroughs. Others, like renal artery reconstruction, have become solidly based on better techniques for diagnostic screening and the insistence on evidence for real pressure gradients. Still others, like the subtotal resection of aneurysms or arterial bypass in the neck, represent logical technical shortcuts that promote simplicity and safety of operation. The virtual disappearance of primary lumbar sympathectomy and extensive endarterectomy speaks for the proved superiority of arterial bypass procedures.

This second edition of *Procedures in Vascular Surgery* follows the outline format of the first in the hope of preserving clarity and brevity. As before, guidelines for diagnosis, indications and contraindications for each procedure, and important intraoperative and postoperative safeguards are set forth. The text and the number of drawings have been considerably expanded to encompass procedural alternatives and step-by-step technical detail. An attempt has been made to present one safe, proved method of carrying through each procedure with attention to avoidance of strategic errors and technical pitfalls. A chapter on intraoperative and postoperative complications has been added.

To Harriet Greenfield, gifted artist, all thanks for her patience and skill in transposing both operating room exposures and the crudest of flat sketches into realistic drawings of depth and character. Furthermore, while preserving her individual style, she has skillfully melded her work into the spirit of the first edition and the drawings by Helen C. Lyman that have been preserved.

Of the many surgeons whose teaching and writing have expanded this field, special recognition is due to Drs. John Homans, Leland S. McKittrick, Robert R. Linton, Frank S. Wheelock, E. A. Edwards, Nathan P. Couch, and Francis D. Moore.

C. C.
R. W.

Boston

Contents

Procedures in vascular surgery

1 Resection and replacement of abdominal aorta for aneurysm

OBJECTIVE

To remove the aneurysm and replace the involved aortic segment with a view to preventing rupture; rarely, to eliminate aortocaval fistula or peripheral embolism.

INDICATIONS

A large aneurysm (over 6 cm. in diameter).

An aneurysm 4 to 6 cm. in diameter in a patient with good cardiac, hepatic, pulmonary, and renal function.

A 4 to 6 cm. aneurysm shown by plain film measurements or echo scan to be enlarging.

A symptomatic aneurysm manifested by pain or hemorrhage, or both.

CONTRAINDICATIONS

In asymptomatic aneurysm: Senility, concomitant disease carrying a life expectancy judged to be less than one year, or mounting renal decompensation. Patients with stable, mild elevations of blood urea nitrogen and creatinine can be carried successfully through aneurysm resection.

In symptomatic aneurysm: None, unless the patient is dying of another disease or if several hours of hypotension with anuria are combined with known prior hypertension or severe pulmonary insufficiency.

PLANNING AND PREPARATION

Asymptomatic Aneurysm: If the diagnosis has been made by physical examination, confirm it by anteroposterior and lateral plain films. Usually, the diagnosis first has been made as a by-product of other x-ray study. If both borders of the aneurysm cannot be clearly outlined on the anteroposterior films and the anterior and posterior walls are not well defined on the lateral view, an echo scan will delineate the size to within 2 to 3 mm.

Perform aortography only if the patient is hypertensive, if the upper border of the pulsating sac is close to the xiphoid process, or if on the anteroposterior plain film the superior rim of the sac *appears* to extend onto the first lumbar vertebra. Even in this last instance, unless the renal arteries clearly come off the sac, there is usually room for insertion of a vascular clamp between the renal arteries and the aneurysm. When the situation is in doubt, oblique or lateral angiograms are helpful.

When angiograms show a noncritical 50 to 60% renal artery stenosis, it should be remembered that division of the aorta just below the renal arteries allows the proximal aorta to move upward. With the renal artery locked down in its bed, this may produce a sharp kink at the plaque and produce severe hypertension. Plans should be made to dissect the affected renal artery free or to place a sidearm bypass off the graft.

Make an excretory urogram to evaluate renal function. Obtain pulmonary function tests or arterial blood gas values, or both, with the patient breathing room air. All patients are made to stop smoking one month prior to admission. Obtain cardiac consultation in all patients. Many should be given digitalis by mouth to a point just short of digitalization prior to the operation.

For the day prior to operation, give clear liquids only, by mouth. At 6:00 A.M. on the morning of the operation, start an intravenous infusion of 5% dextrose in water to provide high urine output levels prior to the induction of anesthesia. A nasogastric tube is placed.

When the patient arrives in the operating room, place a radial artery line, a central venous line, and cardiac monitor leads. Arrange constant bladder drainage so that urine volumes may be recorded at half-hour intervals.

Symptomatic Aneurysm: The operating team should be assembled and the abdomen and groins shaved, prepared, and draped prior to the induction of anesthesia. Sudden hypotension may demand speedy access to the aorta.

OPERATION

Position: Supine. Place both of the patient's arms at his sides to permit assistants easy access. Both groin areas are prepared and draped into the field for possible approach to the common femoral arteries.

Incision: Xiphoid to pubis (Fig. 1-1), left paramedian or midline incision. Carry the upper end invariably into the xiphicostal notch. When the iliac arteries present no special technical problems, the lower half of the incision may be shortened.

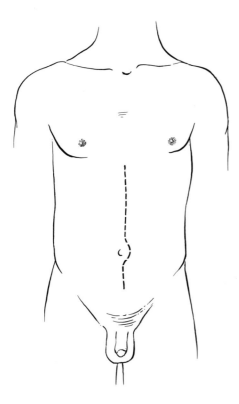

Figure 1-1.   Incision.

Explore the abdomen. Pack the small intestine to the right, the sigmoid to the left, and the transverse colon superiorly (Fig. 1-2).

Resection: In ruptured aneurysm the key to the operation is rapid identification and crossclamping of the aorta just below the left renal vein. Since the aortic pulsation may be feeble and the aorta and all local landmarks obscured by hematoma, this must be done mostly by blunt dissection, aided by suction and manual removal of thrombi. The cupped fingers of the operator's left hand, resting on a large gauze pad, are placed directly over the superior pole of the aneurysm, while with the right hand he dissects open the retroperitoneum and the periaortic tissues. using the apposed tips of a long smooth forceps. By a combination of wiping, blunt dissection with the tip of the closed forceps, sponging, and suction, the left renal vein can be cleaned free and the whitish aorta immediately beneath it scrubbed into full view. One should recall that the left renal vein is retroaortic in 2 to 3% of patients, and in such cases the superior mesenteric artery is the first guide to the location of the renal arteries. If at any point in this dissection further bleeding occurs from the point of rupture, compress shut the neck of the sac with the

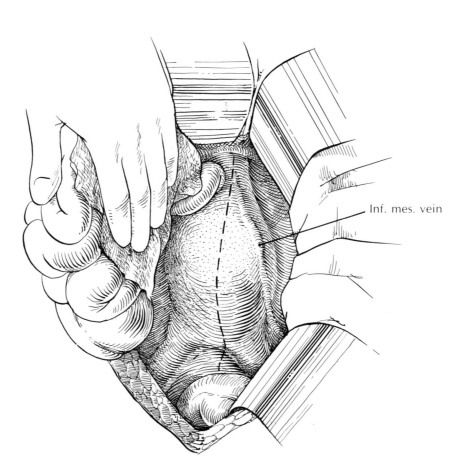

Inf. mes. vein

Figure 1-2.   Packing off intestines.

fingertips of the left hand while continuing to clear the periaortic tissues just above. In this urgent circumstance the central point is the sure identification of the anterior wall of the aorta just below the left renal vein, so that a large vascular clamp can be forced backward onto the aorta from its anterior aspect.

Two other steps are occasionally useful in controlling hemorrhage from a ruptured aneurysm. A tightly folded gauze sponge grasped in a large pulmonary lobe forceps can be firmly directed somewhat from the patient's left, which will compress the aorta above the renal arteries against the spine.

Alternatively the aneurysm can be opened directly with a knife, so that a Foley catheter with a 30-cc. bag can be thrust directly into the suprarenal aorta and the bag rapidly inflated during inflow control by compression.

In elective cases, open the retroperitoneum just to the left of the curve made by the third portion of the duodenum as it overlies the right border of the aneurysm (Fig. 1-2). This opening extends from the left renal vein down the midline of the aneurysm to a point 4 to 5 cm. below the aortic bifurcation. The inferior mesenteric vein will lie to the left of this opening. Retract it with the retroperitoneum to the left. It can be divided and ligated if necessary.

Dissect the waist of the aneurysm laterally in both directions, dividing the inferior mesenteric artery 1 cm. from its aortic takeoff (Fig. 1-3). Carry this dissection exactly to the wall of the vena cava on the right and well short of the origins of the lumbar arteries on the left (Fig. 1-4A, inset). There is little point in trying to clear the left posterolateral wall of the sac; this only results in troublesome venous bleeding. Retract, distort, or compress the sac as little as possible, to avoid the dislodgment of contained thrombus.

As the dissection proceeds to the left renal vein above the upper border of the aneurysm, deepen the peritoneal opening over the aorta through the

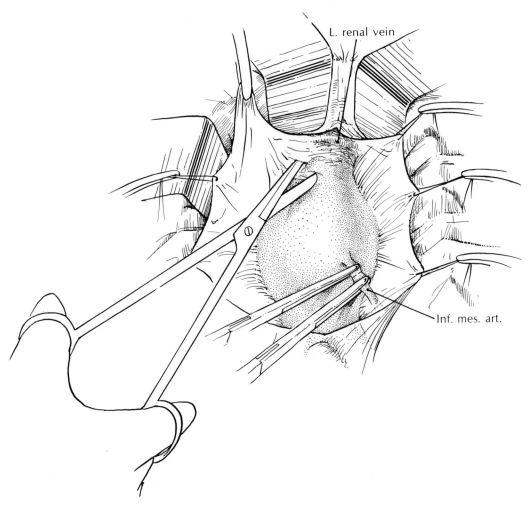

L. renal vein

Inf. mes. art.

Figure 1-3.   Start of aneurysm dissection.

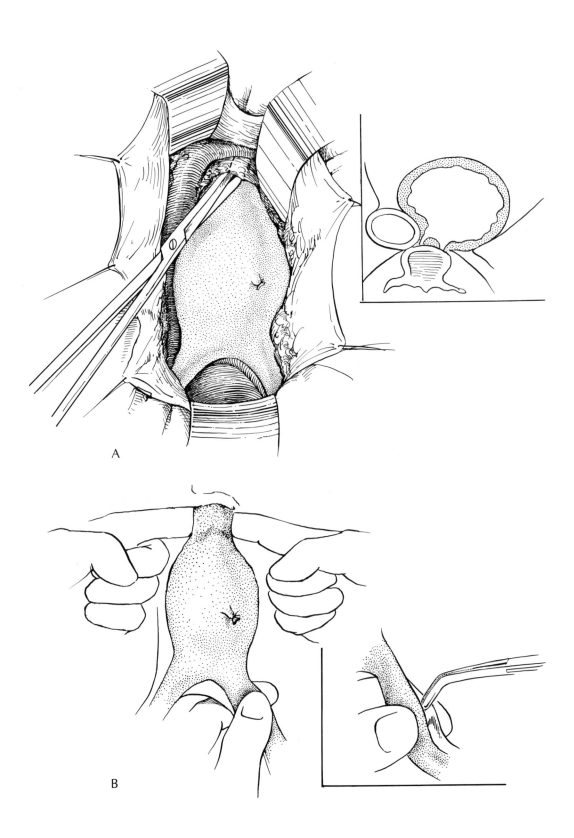

A

B

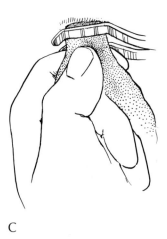

C

Figure 1-4.   (A) Exposure of left renal vein. Extent of lateral dissection (*inset*). (B) Finger behind aneurysm neck. Dissection of left iliac artery and vein (*inset*). (C) Clamping aorta above aneurysm.

underlying fibrous and fatty tissue right over the aorta until actual whitish aortic wall is encountered (Fig. 1-4A). Develop this plane, just outside the adventitia, slowly and carefully in a bright dry field, until the anterior two-thirds of the aortic circumference is cleared free. Place the volar tip of the left index finger directly on the aorta posteromedially and separate away the tissues behind with a burrowing motion. The tip of this finger will identify any intervening lumbar artery, which, if present, must be exposed, ligated, and divided. Do not use hemostatic clips, as they are often wiped loose or pulled off by a retractor tip. Expose and divide strands of fibrous tissue, which sometimes feel at first like lumbar arteries. By keeping the encircling fingertip directly on the adventitia, first on the right and then on the left, injury to large retroaortic and lumbar veins can almost always be avoided (Fig. 1-4B).

If a source of major venous bleeding from behind the aorta is not immediately identified and controlled, pack the area and leave it alone while dissecting free the common iliac arteries. Clamp the aorta in the anteroposterior plane; thus the venous bleeding can easily be dealt with after the aorta is cut across and most of the aneurysm sac removed. Most blood loss in aneurysm resection is of venous origin, and much is unnecessary, since it often stems from premature attempts at control before full exposure is possible. Firm packing for 5 to 10 minutes, by itself, will cut down the rate of venous bleeding very markedly. Major venous hemorrhage, whether from traction avulsion of a branch vein or dissection injury of a lumbar vein, iliac vein, or vena cava, should not be approached by grabs with a right-angled or other hemostatic clamp. This is often not only futile and wasteful of blood, but also enlarges the venous opening. Compress the venous defect and the surrounding tissues with the flat of the fingertips of the left hand while the area is cleared of blood by suction and irrigation. By elevating one finger at a time the operator can demonstrate the location and extent of the venous opening. Most of it can readily be held shut by the tip of the index or middle fingers or both. With the suction tip right on the tissue and the fingertip sliding slightly to one side, visualize the edge of the opening. Using the tips of a large smooth forceps or Allis forceps, gently grasp the entire opening while withdrawing the finger and elevating the vein and surrounding tissues so that an excluding curved vascular clamp can be applied beneath the forceps. Then close the venous opening by a two-bite or running suture.

If the venous opening lies immediately adjacent to adherent iliac artery or aneurysm sac, the preceding maneuver is not feasible. Instead, suture the venous wall to the arterial adventitia and leave this artificial adherence intact when the aneurysm sac is later trimmed away.

The dissection and actual isolation of the common iliac arteries from the corresponding vein are often the most difficult parts of the procedure and the most conducive to venous injury. Adherence of artery to vein increases markedly as one nears the aortic bifurcation, as disease of the artery wall increases, and as the artery becomes more aneurysmal. The least adherence is distal, next to the iliac bifurcation and beyond.

The separation of the common iliac artery from the corresponding vein is most safely done by actually grasping both vessels after preliminary dissection between the thumb and fingers of the left hand, rotating both so that the adherent junction is clearly seen (Fig. 1-4B, inset). Use the tip of a right-angled clamp to burrow under gently, to isolate nonvascular tissue, to draw forcefully like a wedge to split the line of adherence, and to separate the vessels by spreading. Use traction on a tape drawn through the initial small opening beneath the artery to help this opening so that it will admit one finger.

If a large aneurysm of the common iliac artery is present, make no attempt to dissect its deep aspect. Isolate the external iliac artery and carry this dissection as far as feasible, hoping to free up the iliac bifurcation and to gain control of the internal iliac artery. If, because of the bulk of the aneurysm, exposure of this bifurcation is at all difficult, abandon attempts to control hypogastric backflow. Similarly, if there is a significant aneurysm of the hypogastric artery, make no initial attempt to gain distal control of this vessel. In both of these situations the aneurysm involved can be readily dissected after crossclamping the aorta and transecting the vessel concerned. The minor backbleeding from the hypogastric artery can be controlled either by clamping the aneurysm sac shut, by holding a pledget wedged into the mouth of this artery, or by inflating an intraluminal Fogarty catheter. In large, high aneuryms the upper pole of the sac may make visualization and dissection of the left renal vein and proximal aorta difficult without much compression and distortion of the aneurysm. In these situations, clamp the common iliac arteries early to prevent showers of small atheromatous emboli that will cause untreatable distal necrosis.

With the dissection of the aneurysm completed, give 7500 units of heparin intravenously.

Select a Satinsky clamp of suitable size. Arrange for good retraction and clear visualization of the aneurysm neck. Pinch the aorta shut between the thumb in front and the index finger behind, so as to slide the clamp in place just above the aneurysm with the jaws only partly opened and the tips well seen (Fig. 1-4C). Tie a gauze sponge through the handles to prevent the clamp from springing loose. Kelly clamps serve well on the proximal common iliac arteries. They lie well, never slip off, and provide a firm grasp to aid in dissection of the distal artery.

With all clamps in place, open the aneurysm anteriorly with a knife and extend the incision with the scissors from 2 cm. below the upper clamp to the bifurcation below. Grasp the lateral walls in Kocher clamps and scoop out the lining clot. Use pressure on a large, dry gauze pad as a tampon on the lumbar artery mouths. Of the six or eight in the field, usually only two or three will backbleed significantly. Deep near and far sutures of 3-0 silk on strong, large needles are used to control these friable and often calcific ostia (Fig. 1-5A). At this point trim away most of the aortic sac (Fig. 1-5B and C).

Pass the index finger behind the aorta again, but below the clamp, and divide the aortic cuff carefully at the level of the upper end of the aortotomy—no higher—with the scissors (Fig. 1-5D). The tongue of the aortic wall posteriorly and next to the vena cava is then sewed shut with a deeply placed running 0 catgut suture (Fig. 1-5E). This stops all oozing from the cut edge, closes all lumbar arteries, and often improves hemostasis greatly.

Preparing for Graft: With the upper clamp now free, clear the aortic cuff circumferentially, often right up to the renal arteries. The goal here is to develop the best available segment of aorta. Place a second Satinsky clamp above the first one. Now remove the first clamp and trim away another centimeter or two of friable, crumbly aorta, leaving a 1.5-cm. cuff of sound artery. Select a bifurcation graft whose various calibers best approximate those of the host arteries. The tightly woven grafts, which do not require preclotting, have real advantages in this setting, in which late thrombosis is almost unknown. In ruptured aneurysm, in which clotting factors are often depleted, the tightly woven grafts are ideal. Pull the crimp out and trim the aortic segment suitably short.

Cylinder grafts sutured blindly through the back wall at either end inside

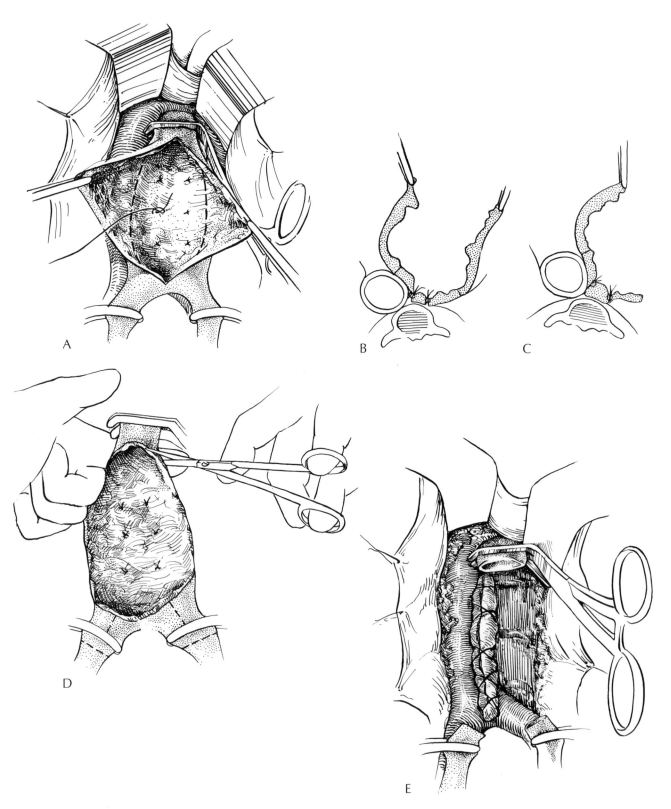

Figure 1-5. (*A*) Opening and partial excision of aneurysm. Suturing off lumbar arteries. (*B*) Extent of cross-section, indicating excision of aneurysm wall. (*C*) Further excision of sac. (*D*) Transecting neck of aneurysm. (*E*) Securing cut edge of aneurysm wall.

the opened aneurysm sac may have a place as a time-saver in ruptured aneurysm. Otherwise, they have drawbacks. A suture leak is hard to find and harder to repair. The aorta at the upper suture line is often not sound. Stenotic or aneurysmal iliac segments are left behind. Blind suture lines are difficult to certify.

Aortic Anastomosis: Many good techniques have been devised for end-to-end suture of a prosthetic graft to the divided aorta. A generally leakproof method is described.

   The aortic clamp is rocked up by an assistant, and two lateral mattress sutures are placed exactly 180 degrees from each other (Fig. 1-6A). Any difference in circumference between graft and aorta is distributed equally between the two hemicircles. Take sutures 5 to 6 mm. deep into both graft and aorta to include a 5-mm. width. Tie both sutures down. This everts the suture line at those points. Large bites of graft and artery well compressed by suture tension are more hemostatic than are many shallow sutures. With the graft turned up over the patient's chest, sew the posterior row over and over from left to right, passing the needle through both aorta and graft in one bite for each stitch (Fig. 1-6B). It is only rarely necessary to pick up the edge of either the graft or aorta with the forceps. Push these everted edges into proper

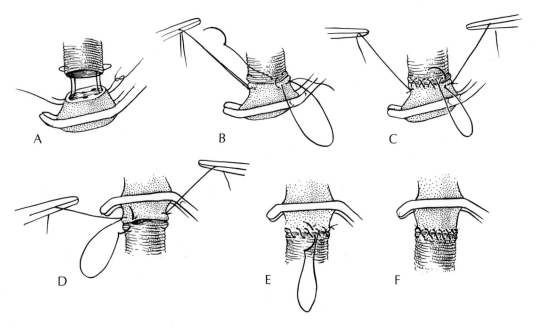

Figure 1-6.   (A) Aortic suture line—lateral mattress sutures. (B) Posterior suture line. (C) Running back the posterior suture line. (D) Starting the anterior suture line. (E) Running back the second row. (F) Completed anastomosis.

apposition, with the tips of the closed forceps indenting one edge of the suture line and the tip of the needle the other. With the first assistant "tagging" the suture, and each stitch pulled tight against the tip of the forceps, the eversion is easily maintained. Tie this first suture to the standing part of the right-hand mattress suture and then carry it back in shallower bites, between the first sutures, to the point of origin, and tie it to itself (Fig. 1-6C). This creates a very tight cross-stitch that rarely leaks.

The posterior row is now inspected from within to be sure that the anterior wall of the graft has not been caught in any prior suture.

Turn the clamp down so that the aortic cuff and the graft lie in their ultimate position. Using the right-hand suture, suture the front row from right to left (Fig. 1-6D) and back again to create a similar cross-stitch (Fig. 1-6E and F). The second suture line takes only 2 to 3 minutes in each case, and it often prevents troublesome leaks that would require reapplication of the aortic clamp.

Test the upper suture line with saline injected under pressure or by grasping the prosthesis tightly just below the anastomosis and partially opening the upper clamp. Then strip and suction all blood out of the graft.

Iliac Artery Anastomosis: Further dissect the left iliac artery to just below its bifurcation and apply a single vascular clamp just below that level, taking care that the arteries lie naturally, without twisting. Trim away the crushed proximal end. Remove the clamp momentarily to demonstrate free backbleeding. If backbleeding is feeble, use the Fogarty catheter to clear out all clots. Trim away the left limb of the graft so that slight tension is placed as the first mattress suture is tied. Most aorta-to-common femoral grafts are too tight; most aorta-to-common iliac grafts are too loose.

The simplest graft-to-iliac artery anastomosis is made with both cut at right angles, assuming that the iliac lumen is of sufficient caliber. The operator unites the two with a mattress suture placed at the point on the ultimate circumference that is farthest from him (Fig. 1-7A). Traction on that suture will anteriorly rotate the site for the next bite into excellent view so that he can suture the front row with a good look into each open lumen (Fig. 1-7B). Again pass the needle through both artery and graft in one bite for each stitch, using the tips of the forceps as a counterforce on the graft right next to each point at which the needle will emerge.

When the suture line is half done, pass the standing part of the original suture behind the anastomosis and rotate the clamps so that the posterior half of the suture line comes into full view (Fig. 1-7C). The same over-and-over suture is continued to the point of origin and tied to itself (Fig. 1-7D and E).

When the iliac artery is small, or considerable disproportion exists between graft and artery, an oblique anastomosis at 45 degrees, or slightly less, is ideal (Fig. 1-8A). Make cuts in the coronal plane; then, of the two mattress sutures joining the two ends of the ellipses together, one will lie directly posterior and

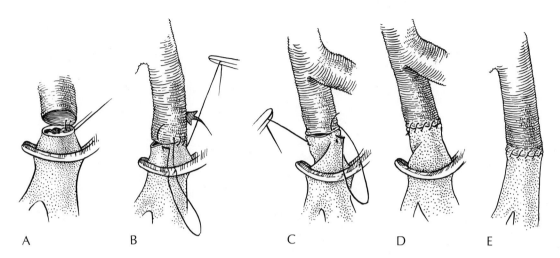

Figure 1-7.   (A) Left iliac suture line, transverse anastomosis. (B) Completing the first half. (C) Bringing the back half into view. (D) Tying to the original suture. (E) Completed anastomosis.

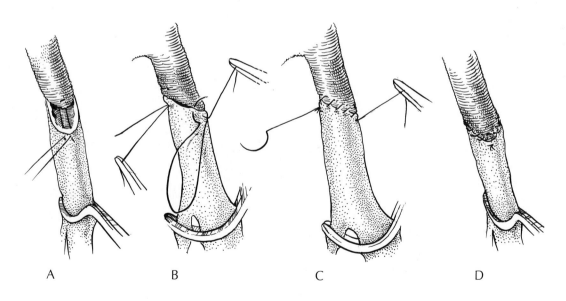

Figure 1-8.   (A) Oblique iliac anastomosis, first two sutures. (B) Rotation to suture right side. (C) Tying to posterior suture. (D) Completed anastomosis.

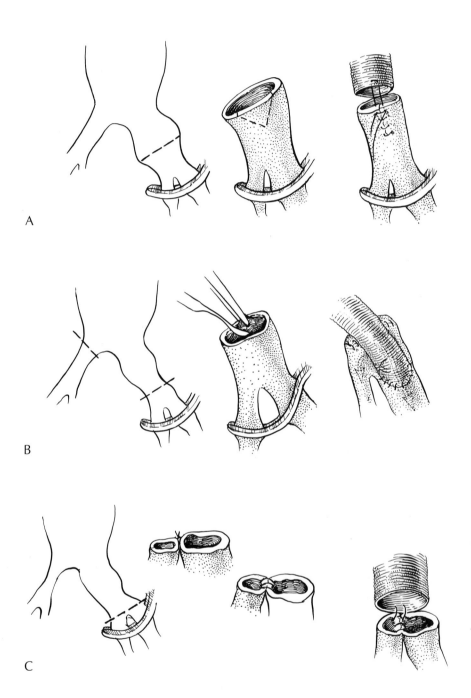

Figure 1-9.   (A) V-excision and anastomosis. (B) Oversewing common iliac artery and anastomosis to external iliac. (C) Anastomosis to recreated iliac bifurcation.

the other directly anterior. By rotating graft and artery only 90 degrees, each suture line can be brought anteriorly for easy suturing (Fig. 1-8B, C, and D).

When the distal third of the common iliac artery is too large for the graft, a V-excision permits tailoring to fit (Fig. 1-9A). If the distal common iliac artery is very thickened and calcified, and the plaque extends well down into the external iliac so that endarterectomy is not feasible, oversew the common iliac and carry out end-to-side anastomosis to the external iliac (Fig. 1-9B). In order to pass needles through the calcific wall of the common iliac artery, it may be necessary to bite out a rim of sclerotic plaque prior to oversewing. Here, there is no concern about dissection under a flap, as blood flow will be coming up from below.

When both the internal and external iliac arteries must be cut across, a new bifurcation must be created (Fig. 1-9C).

When the suture line is completed, briefly flush the aortic stump and graft via the right limb of the graft while blocking access of blood to the left (Fig. 1-10). Then test the aortic anastomosis with saline injected up the right limb. Place a Kelly clamp high on the right limb of the graft, and remove the clamps from the left iliac limb of the graft and from the iliac arteries. Remove the

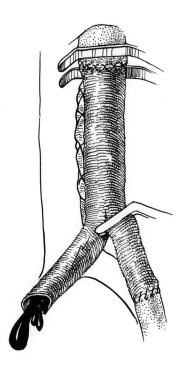

Figure 1-10.   Graft being flushed.

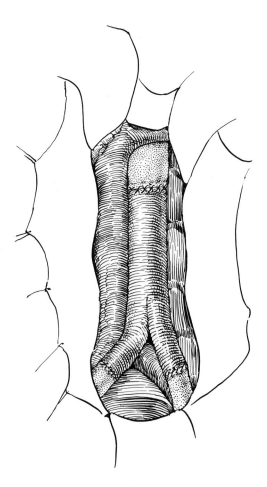

Figure 1-11.   Graft completed.

aortic clamp slowly or, even better, control the flow through the graft with the left hand as the clamp is loosened. One has no sense of the volume of flow through a partially opened clamp.

Leaks between sutures should not be repaired under full arterial pressure. This is not only wasteful of blood, but also the artery is often cut by the needle and the bite taken is wider than the others, making for a cutting effect as the suture is tied. These bites should usually be somewhat smaller than the others (at times only adventitial), and the suture should be tied with the artery under very low or no pressure. On the other hand, leaks should be repaired expeditiously. If mainstream clamps are reapplied many times, clotting in the graft may result.

Following completion of the anastomosis, perform the second iliac anastomosis in a similar manner (Fig. 1-11). Take 15 to 20 minutes to ensure complete hemostasis. Every nook and cranny of the retroperitoneal dissection must be irrigated and carefully inspected for bleeding points. Protamine sulfate in suitable doses is usually given. Every effort is made to ensure that the patient will not require subsequent exploration for bleeding.

Close the retroperitoneum very carefully. In the suturing, avoid the ureters, inferior mesenteric vein, vena cava, and duodenum. If chronic obstructive pulmonary disease is severe, use a gastrostomy. Retention sutures in the abdominal wall are used in every case.

2   *Thromboendarterectomy of the aortoiliac segment for obliterative arteriosclerosis*

OBJECTIVE

To transport mainstream arterial flow to the deprived tissues below the block.

INDICATIONS

Disabling arterial insufficiency in the lower extremities. In older people, moderate intermittent claudication alone is not an indication, but in younger people it usually is. Make the decision on the basis of functional and economic disability. The operation does not alter the disease process.

Accompanying renal insufficiency or arterial hypertension due to renal artery stenosis resulting from the aortic arteriosclerotic process.

Wide patency of the external iliac arteries. These must be of good caliber and show minimal arteriosclerotic involvement.

Although thromboendarterectomy was formerly widely used for blocks extending below the iliac bifurcation, it is now chosen in preference to aortoiliac bypass only when significant occlusive disease is limited to the aortic and common iliac segments. In longer blocks the advantage it affords of avoiding insertion of foreign material is offset by the length of the dissection, the increased operation time, and the resultant failure of ejaculation in some males. In over 30% of patients, aortoiliac blocks are so extensive that thromboendarterectomy is impossible to accomplish satisfactorily, even by prolonged efforts.

CONTRAINDICATIONS

Progressive renal insufficiency of a type that will not be improved by the operative maneuver.

Senility.

Any concomitant disease with a limited prognosis.

PLANNING AND PREPARATION

Perform aortography or arteriography to determine the location and extent of aortoiliac disease and, in hypertensive patients, of renal artery disease as well.

Prepare the groins as well as the abdomen, for it may be necessary to change to bypass.

Details of preparation are as for aneurysm, except that no arterial line for monitoring is usually necessary.

OPERATION

Position: Supine.

Incision and Exposures: Left paramedian, xiphoid to lower abdomen (Fig. 2-1). Obtain abdominal exposure as in the approach to aneurysm (Figs. 1-2 and 2-2A).

Assessment of Arteries: First determine the operability of the lower segments by dissecting both iliac bifurcations, including on each side 2 cm. of each of the three vessels involved. Place a right-angled clamp behind each of these segments to permit palpation through the wall onto the clamp; this will give a clear appreciation of the distribution of the arterial thickening and the caliber of the lumen (Fig. 2-2B).

There are two problem areas in aortoiliac thromboendarterectomy. The first, as mentioned, involves the status of the external iliac arteries. If these are found to be of smaller caliber and more diseased than indicated on the arteriograms, shift over to aortofemoral bypass forthwith. The second problem involves the iliac artery bifurcations, where careful management is critical to the success of the operation. Two situations may confront the operator. First, if the heavy intimal plaque of the common iliac artery continues uniformly down the external iliac, and perhaps the hypogastric, albeit with adequate caliber, abandon the thought of endarterectomy involving this bifurcation. In this case, divide the common iliac with a sharp blade straight across just above the bifurcation in order not to disturb the distal intima. Then reanastomose it end to end to the endarterectomized common iliac segment (Fig. 2-3). This maneuver guarantees that the distal intima is completely sutured down circumferentially. The second, and ideal, situation is seen when the common iliac intimal plaque abruptly thins down in a tooth-root manner to virtually normal intima above, at, or only 8 or 10 mm. into, the external and internal iliac arteries, a situation exactly like that seen in the stenotic carotid artery bifurcation and often in the deep femoral artery. This pattern is most amenable to a clean endarterectomy.

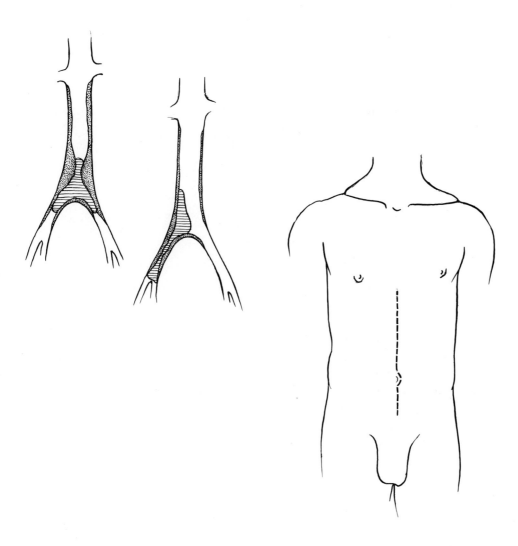

Figure 2-1.   Diagram of disease, bilateral and unilateral.

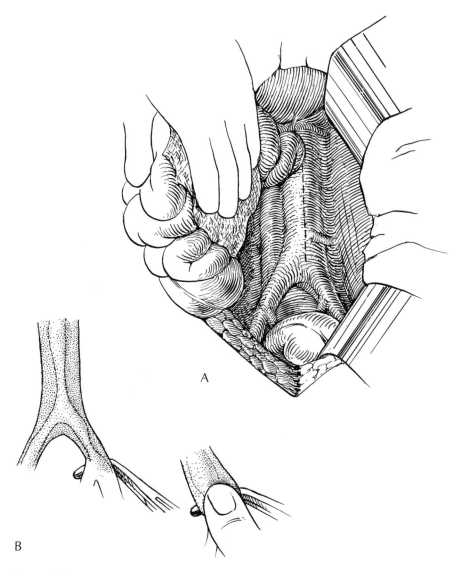

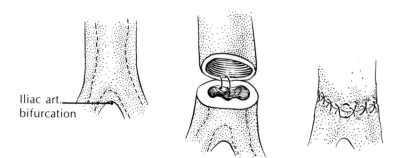

Iliac art. bifurcation

Figure 2-2. (A) Exposure of the aorta and iliac arteries. (B) External arterial assessment.

Figure 2-3. Anastomosis of endarterectomized common iliac segment to transected distal segment.

Operative Steps: Dissect the abdominal aorta for a few centimeters near the proposed upper limit of endarterectomy. Avoid division of the inferior mesenteric artery and the large lumbar branches if they are patent and if their division is unnecessary. Apply temporary occluding clamps to those undivided branches communicating with the proposed open aortic segment (Fig. 2-4).

Clear the common iliac arteries down to the level of the prior dissection, using gentle elevation by traction tapes to help free these arteries from underlying veins.

Give 7500 units of heparin intravenously just after the dissection and 7500 units per hour thereafter during the procedure.

Perform thromboendarterectomy of the upper segment of the abdominal aorta and carry it down to the point previously selected (Fig. 2-5). If disease

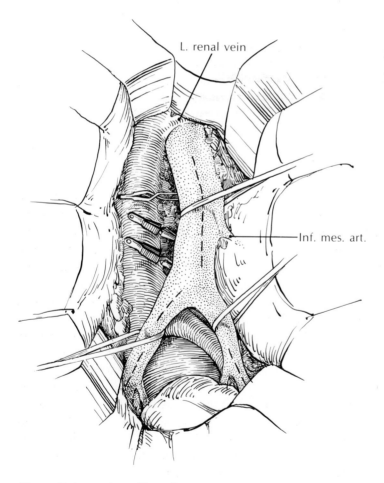

Figure 2-4.   Aortoiliac dissection.

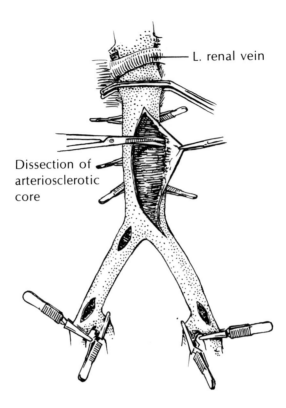

— L. renal vein

Dissection of
arteriosclerotic
core

Figure 2-5.   Start of thromboendarterectomy.

extends to the renal arteries, both of these should be dissected, as well as the aorta just above them. Do the thromboendarterectomy by carrying the aortic incision upward to within 3 cm. of the renal arteries (Fig. 2-6) and removing the arteriosclerotic material; use digital compression of the upper aorta above the renal arteries during removal of the aortic clamp (Fig. 2-7). It is important to deal with partial as well as complete blocks at that time. Momentarily clamp the renal arteries, which should be previously cleared with this in mind, in order to avoid renal embolism during this maneuver.

Close the upper thromboendarterectomy incision with a double layer of sutures down to the lowest open large branch. Move the aortic clamp below this branch to allow some improved circulation while the lower part of the thromboendarterectomy incision is closed. It is especially important that the circulation to a limb that had pulses before the operation be reopened at the earliest opportunity. Manage the lower end of the reconstruction in accordance with considerations outlined on page 20. Figure 2-3 depicts the transection endarterectomy method. Figure 2-8 shows closure of all arteriotomies, the lower end being managed in the traditional manner.

Close the peritoneum and abdomen as in Chapter 1.

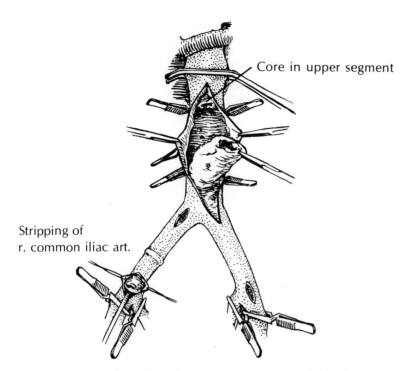

Core in upper segment

Stripping of
r. common iliac art.

Figure 2-6.   Thromboendarterectomy—core mobilized.

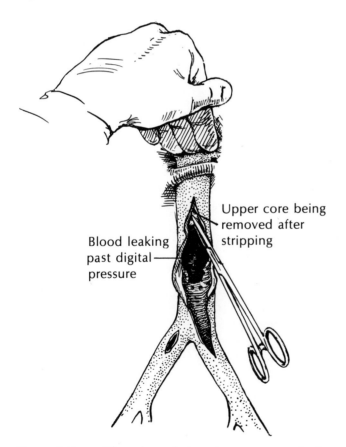

Blood leaking
past digital
pressure

Upper core being
removed after
stripping

Figure 2-7.   Thromboendarterectomy—removal of upper core.

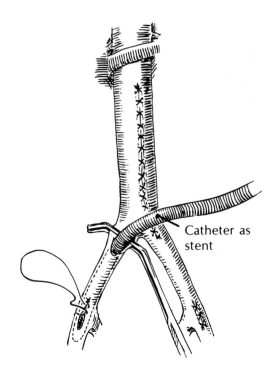

Catheter as
stent

Figure 2-8.   Arteriotomy closure.

NOTES ON MANAGEMENT OF ASSOCIATED
RENAL ARTERY STENOSIS

Renal artery encroachment or involvement, when present, follows three general patterns, each managed in a different way.

Aortic Thrombosis with Encroachment on Renal Arteries but No Stenosis or
Hypertension: See Figure 2-9A.

   Dissect both renal arteries for 2 cm. and the aorta to just above these
arteries.

   Apply a single clamp above all clot and across the aorta and both renal
arteries, then perform endarterectomy.

   Curette out the clot. Irrigate the segment. Close the upper 2 cm. of the
aortotomy. Move the clamp down.

Aortic Thrombosis with Atheromatous Stenosis of Renal Arteries and Hyper-
tension: See Figure 2-9B.

   Dissect both renal arteries for 2 cm. and the aorta up to the superior
mesenteric artery. Apply three clamps and perform a long aortotomy to just

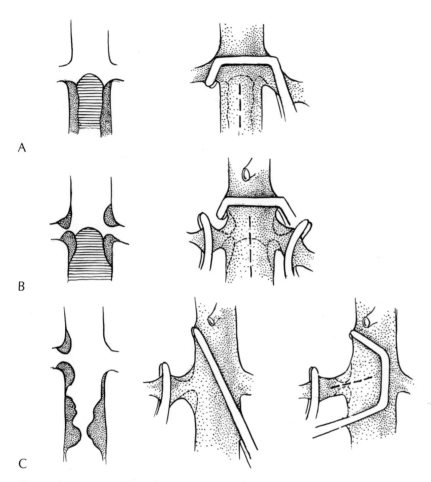

Figure 2-9.   (*A*) Renal artery encroachment, no stenosis. (*B*) Bilateral renal artery stenosis. (*C*) Unilateral renal artery stenosis.

above the renal arteries. Wide intraaortic exposure is vital to good visualization of the renal artery ostia.

Remove the clot and perform endarterectomy on both renal arteries from within.

Close 3 cm. of the aortotomy and move the aortic clamp down.

No High Aortic Thrombosis, Unilateral Renal Artery Stenosis, and Hypertension: See Figure 2-9C.

Dissect the involved renal artery for 3 cm. and the aorta for 1 cm. above both renal vessels.

Using either one of two possible techniques (Fig. 2-9C), clamp across the aorta and above only one renal artery. Place the arteriotomy over the origin of the renal artery. Allow an ample length of arteriotomy through which to dissect the plaque in order to avoid injury to the back wall of the artery.

3 Aortoiliac and aortofemoral bypass for obliterative arteriosclerosis

OBJECTIVE

To restore central aortic pressure to the common femoral artery.

INDICATIONS

Disabling arterial insufficiency in the lower extremities from aortoiliac stenosis. In older people, moderate intermittent claudication alone is not an indication, but in younger people, it usually is. The decision is made on the basis of functional and economic disability. The operation does not alter the disease process.

Occasional coexisting renal artery stenosis causing hypertension. This can be dealt with at the same operation (see Chaps. 2 and 13).

Patency or correctable stenosis of the deep femoral artery.

CONTRAINDICATIONS

The absence of patency of both the superficial and deep femoral arteries (very rare).

Senility.

Any concomitant disease with a limited prognosis.

Renal insufficiency of a type that will not be improved by the operation.

PLANNING AND PREPARATION

Perform aortography to prove the presence of significant aortoiliac stenosis, to delineate the extent of disease in or just below the renal arteries, and to show the patency of the common femoral or deep femoral arteries or of both.

OPERATION

Position: Supine.

29

Incision and Exposure: If the common femoral artery is to be the site of the lower anastomosis, make the groin incision(s) over the femoral artery, about 8 cm. long, with the upper end at the inguinal ligament (Fig. 3-1). However, if the aortogram shows that the distal external iliac arteries are open and appropriate for the destination of the bypass and that there is no deep femoral stenosis, make short, oblique incisions parallel to and just above the inguinal ligaments (Fig. 3-1). Rarely, both incisions will be made, for example, when the external iliac on exposure is found to be considerably more diseased than was suggested in the angiogram. Always leave an intact skin bridge over the inguinal ligament.

The oblique incision above the inguinal ligament, when used, is deepened through the fascia transversalis, at which point the intact peritoneum is swept upward. Free up a 5-cm. length of external iliac artery and begin the lower end of the retroperitoneal tunnel by blunt dissection directly along the anterior wall of the artery.

The more usual common femoral dissection will include about 5 cm. of that artery and 2.5 cm. of both the superficial and the deep femoral arteries (Fig. 3-2).

If endarterectomy of the common femoral or deep femoral artery is necessary, defer it until after the aortic anastomosis. Make the tunnel under the inguinal ligament under good vision and by slowly and gently spreading the tissues with a full-length clamp so that the epigastric or circumflex iliac veins will not be injured. The index finger both dissects and ensures that the proper plane is maintained right on the artery.

Make the abdominal incision in a manner similar to that described in Chapter 2, but do not extend it lower in the abdomen than the midpoint between the umbilicus and the pubis.

Expose the aorta exactly as in Chapter 2, but dissect only that segment between the left renal vein and the inferior mesenteric artery. Divide and ligate two sets of lumbar arteries so that an 8-cm. length of aorta is mobilized (Fig. 3-2). The aortic wall above the inferior mesenteric artery is considerably less subject to atheromatous change than that below.

Any unusually large lumbar artery should be preserved and controlled with a bulldog clamp in case it should carry a special supply to the anterior spinal artery of the cord.

Make the retroperitoneal tunnels that join the aortic exposure with the dissections below by working the index fingers of both hands toward each other. A large, blunt, slightly curved aneurysm clamp is often helpful both in creating the tunnel and in drawing a tape through it to facilitate the later passage of the same clamp. The ureter will move with the peritoneum, ultimately to lie anterior to the graft.

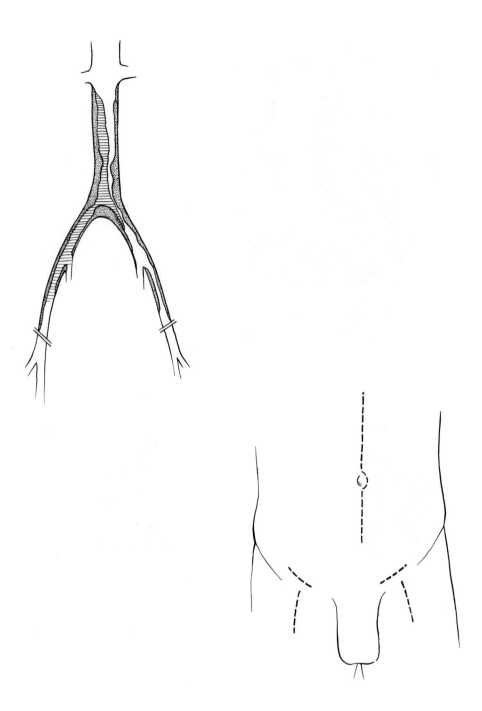

Figure 3-1.   Incision and diagram of disease.

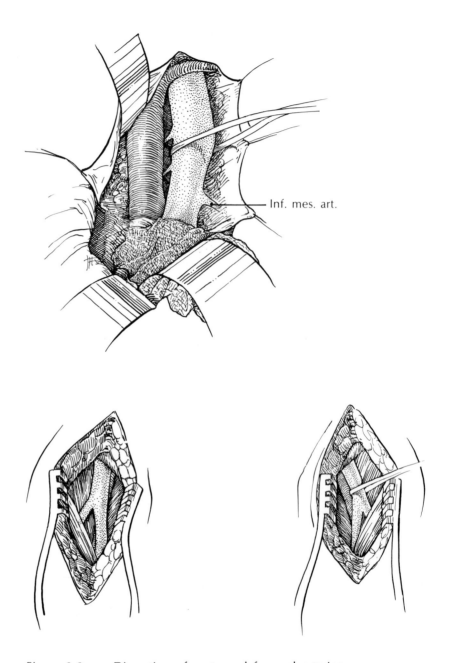

Inf. mes. art.

Figure 3-2.   Dissection of aorta and femoral arteries.

Give 7500 units of heparin.

Now place two clamps on the aorta (Fig. 3-3), one just below the left renal vein and one just above, or at times including, the inferior mesenteric artery. Two clamps are much better than one large J-clamp, because either one can be loosened separately for flushing or to release entrapped clot or thickened plaque. There is a strong tendency to place these clamps too closely together, cramping the long arteriotomy needed to accommodate a large bifurcation graft cut across at 45 degrees. Remember also that any arteriotomy should stop 1 cm. short of a clamp to allow ample room for placing the end suture.

Preparation of Aorta for Graft.   Open the aorta between the clamps and perform any thromboendarterectomy necessary to provide proper inflow to the graft and remove laminated clot. Clear the segment above the clamp by flushing. Leave enough substance to the wall to allow firm suture. Compulsive endarterectomy will ultimately thin out the edges of the arteriotomy, possibly promoting late false aneurysm arising at the anastomosis.

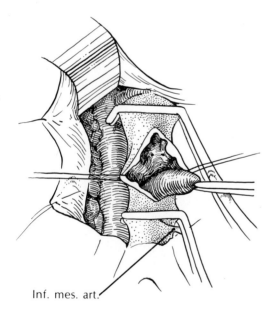

Inf. mes. art.

Figure 3-3.   Preparation of aorta.

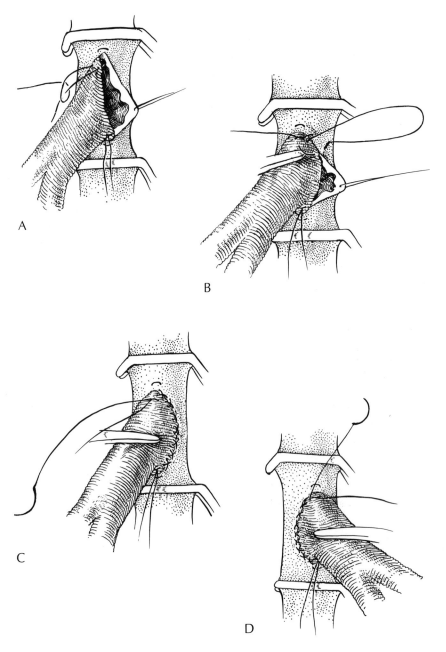

Figure 3-4.   (A) Mattress sutures outlining anastomosis. (B) Running the suture down the left side. (C) Completing the left-side cross-stitch. (D) Completed aortic anastomosis.

Cut the graft at 45 degrees no more than 5 cm. above its bifurcation. After placing stay sutures at the edges of the aortotomy, place a mattress suture through the graft and through each end of the aortotomy (Fig. 3-4A) and tie these down. Run the left side of the anastomosis down from above in an over-and-over manner (Fig. 3-4B) and tie with two throws to the standing part of the second mattress suture. Run the first needle back up the left side in a slightly shallower cross-stitch between bites and tie to the suture of origin (Fig. 3-4C). The right side of the anastomosis can be run down and back again with the original needle (Fig. 3-4D) or run up from below using the second mattress suture.

In this suturing, large (5- to 6-mm.) bites of both graft and artery are taken. Pick up the cut edges of the graft or artery in the forceps as rarely as possible. Use the tip of the closed forceps to indent the graft against the wall of the artery at a point just deep to where the needle will emerge. This everts the suture line, adjusts the graft and aortic edges into well-seen apposition, and supports both graft and aortic wall against the thrust of the needle. Thus, suturing of the aorta from without in is perfectly feasible. When suturing from the graft out through the aortic wall, the needle tip is used to evert and position the graft while the forceps supports the aortic wall next to the point of emergence of the needle.

Test the anastomosis with saline and close any significant suture-line leaks. Draw the right limb of the graft down through the prepared tunnel, using a large, slightly curved clamp and guarding against twisting of the limb (Fig. 3-5).

If the lower end of the bypass is to be at the common femoral level, the decision for or against any endarterectomy of the common femoral artery or deep femoral artery must now be made. Usually the anterior wall of the common femoral artery is soft, and endarterectomy of this segment should not be done unless marked narrowing of the common femoral artery itself is noted on the angiogram and is demonstrable as a dense circumferential plaque on exposure of the vessel. If stenosis of the deep femoral artery is evident on the arteriogram, carefully palpate its first 3 cm., pressing the

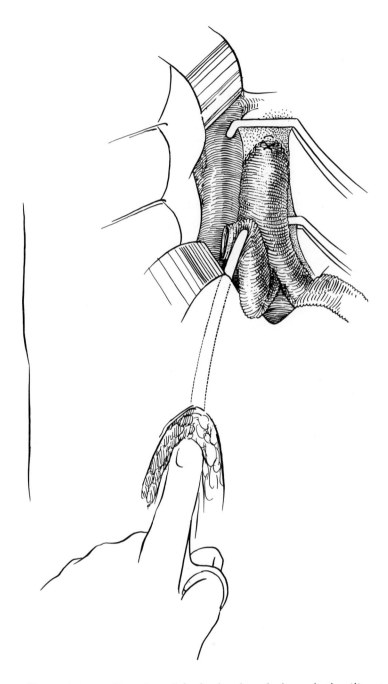

Figure 3-5.   Drawing right limb of graft through the iliac tunnel.

arterial wall against an underlying right-angled clamp. This will demonstrate that the ostial plaque thins out abruptly at 1 cm. or so (Fig. 3-6A), or that the intimal thickening continues on down the vessel. In the first circumstance, which is often signaled by a poststenotic dilatation of the deep femoral artery, open the common femoral artery via a 3-cm. arteriotomy extending just beyond its bifurcation onto the superficial femoral artery (Fig. 3-6B). Place stay sutures at the edges of the arteriotomy (Fig. 3-6C). Perform endarterectomy by finding the easiest plane at one end of the arteriotomy and running the dissector around both sides from there (Fig. 3-6D). Using a right-angled clamp as a blunt dissector near the upper end of the arteriotomy, free up the core circumferentially above the deep femoral branch and cut it off as high as possible with small plastic scissors (Fig. 3-6E). In a similar fashion, dissect around the core as it enters the superficial femoral artery. Usually this core must be cut off. Now the core can easily be freed right down to the stump lying in the mouth of the deep femoral artery (Fig. 3-6E).

The 360-degree view of this stump now available makes possible its gentle blunt dissection and removal, together with the entire common femoral core. Establish the proper dissection plane first in the anterior wall of the deep femoral artery, where visualization is perfect. Develop this plane around posteriorly with great care in order not to perforate the adventitia. After removal of the deep femoral core, run the tip of a Kelly clamp well into the lumen as that vascular clamp is removed. Demonstrate the absence of any intimal shelf by palpation of the Kelly clamp through the artery wall.

Tack down the divided cuff of the superficial femoral branch only if flow is to be restored to that artery (Fig. 3-6F).

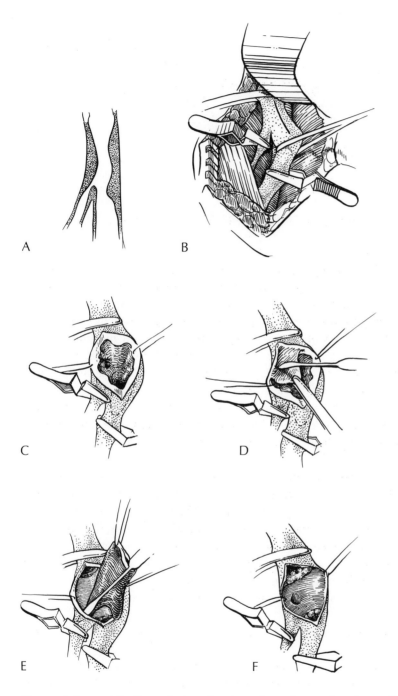

Figure 3-6.   (*A*) Stenosis localized to deep femoral ostium. (*B*) Common femoral arteriotomy. (*C*) Stay sutures, aiding visualization. (*D*) Beginning the endarterectomy. (*E*) Freeing the core from the deep femoral artery. (*F*) Completed endarterectomy.

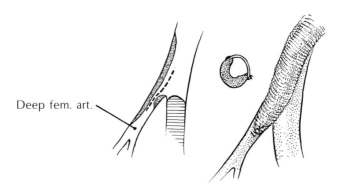

Deep fem. art.

Figure 3-7.   Using the graft to enlarge the deep femoral artery.

If the intimal thickening continues on down the deep femoral artery but the ostium is narrow, carry the arteriotomy in the common femoral down through this ostium to increase the caliber by the patch effect of the graft (Fig. 3-7).

After pulling out most of the crimp, adjust the tension on the right limb of the graft so that there will be no buckling or tortuosity of the limb, yet no tension on the anastomosis. Trim this limb at a 45-degree angle. Place a single mattress suture to hold the graft at the upper end of the arteriotomy. This anastomosis can be carried around the entire arteriotomy with one suture, or a second mattress stitch can be placed at the lower end of the arteriotomy and each side sutured with a different stitch. The latter method ensures a perfect fit of the graft to the artery, but it makes more blind suturing necessary.

If the aortic clamps have never been removed for flushing, this should be done, with the right limb of the graft clamped at its takeoff to allow any clots or debris to pass down the free left limb. Otherwise, remove the femoral clamps first, allowing the graft to fill in a retrograde direction. Clamp the left limb of the graft at its takeoff and milk any blood out of this limb. Remove the lower aortic clamp and then the upper one. Pressure-pack the anastomoses to control tiny stitch hole leaks. Repair any larger leaks with the upper aortic clamp reapplied or with the anastomosis squeezed tightly shut with the fingers.

Draw the left limb of the graft down through its tunnel and complete that anastomosis (Fig. 3-8).

Concomitant lumbar sympathectomy is unnecessary when the femorotibial arteries are relatively normal and strong pedal pulsations can be expected to follow the aortoiliac operation.

When the superficial femoral arteries are obstructed, bilateral lumbar sympathectomy is desirable, not only to enhance flow through the graft by reducing peripheral resistance, but also to increase skin blood flow over the

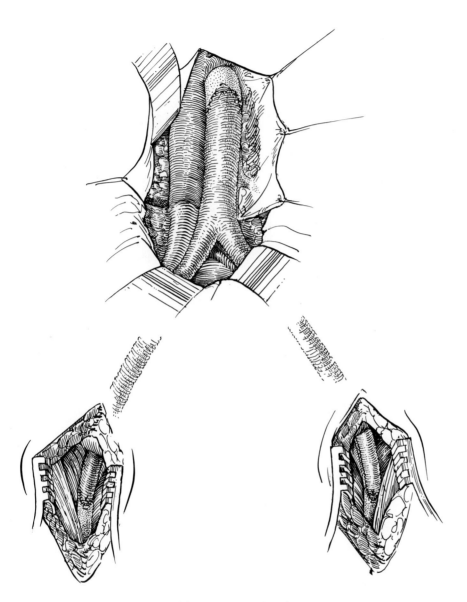

Figure 3-8.   Aortofemoral bypass completed.

feet and toes. If there is any reason to shorten the operation, or if the lumbar sympathetic chain cannot be easily found, it is not mandatory.

The left lumbar chain is easily found at the L3 to L4 level by running the fingertips back and forth in the coronal plane over the anterolateral aspect of these vertebral bodies just under the left edge of the aorta. Much like the vas deferens in the spermatic cord, the chain can be felt against the bone as an easily rolled, firm cord. Pick the chain up in a nerve hook, follow it in both directions, looking for confirming rami communicantes or ganglia, and re- move a 3- to 4-cm. length (see Chap. 12), preferably including two ganglia.

To secure a segment of the right chain, dissect the right side of the vena cava at the same level. Retract the vena cava to the left and palpate for the chain against the right anterolateral aspect of the same vertebrae.

If the lower end of the bypass is to be at the external iliac artery level, draw a 4-cm. loop of that vessel into a curve of a vascular clamp and make a 2-cm. arteriotomy in the anterior wall. Adjust the tension on the corresponding graft limb so that it is neither tight nor redundant, cut at a 45-degree angle, and carry out the end-to-side anastomosis.

If any undue ooze is present, give 50 to 75 mg. of protamine sulfate intravenously.

Close as described in Chapter 1.

4 Axillofemoral and femorofemoral bypass for obliterative arteriosclerosis

INDICATIONS FOR AXILLOFEMORAL BYPASS

Rest pain or gangrene of sufficient extent to threaten the lower extremity.

Sepsis in, or failure of, a prior aortoiliac reconstruction.

Associated disease of sufficient severity to render the patient a high risk for the direct transabdominal approach to the aorta or common iliac arteries.

Unilateral or bilateral aortoiliac occlusion.

If the common femoral artery on either side has been the site of prior operation, or if future femoropopliteal bypass is a possibility, the lower anastomosis may be done to the external iliac just above the inguinal ligament, provided the mouth of the deep femoral artery has been shown by oblique arteriograms to be widely patent.

CONTRAINDICATIONS TO AXILLOFEMORAL BYPASS

None of the conditions listed under "Indications" present.

The long-term patency of axillofemoral grafts is not so high as that with other methods of restoring circulation to the iliofemoral arterial system. It is therefore not used for intermittent claudication alone, even of an advanced degree.

INDICATIONS FOR FEMOROFEMORAL BYPASS

Rest pain, or gangrene that threatens the lower extremity.

Disabling intermittent claudication.

The femorofemoral technique is preferred to the axillofemoral for unilateral aortoiliac disease.

As the passage of time reveals that the patency of the femorofemoral bypass persists for intervals comparable to those following aortofemoral bypass, more surgeons are choosing femorofemoral over aortofemoral grafting on less rigid indications.

CONTRAINDICATIONS TO FEMOROFEMORAL BYPASS

It is important that no stenosis or combination of stenoses sufficient to produce a pressure gradient at rest or on exercise exist in the "good" iliac system, lest creation of the bypass produce a "steal."

PLANNING AND PREPARATION

Same as described in Chapter 3.

For the axillofemoral bypass, plan to use a 10-mm. plastic prosthesis. The biologic advantages of the autogenous vein for arterial replacement are offset by the length of vein and the time of preparation required, together with the likelihood of inadequate caliber.

For femorofemoral bypass, choose either an 8-mm. or 10-mm. prosthesis. Since these short grafts rarely fail in themselves and their patency record is impressive, most surgeons have ceased to use veins for this operation.

The routines of preoperative skin preparation, medications, and other measures are similar to those described in Chapter 2. Either type of bypass can be done under local anesthesia, but since it is tedious for the patient, use it only where general or spinal anesthesia is strongly contraindicated.

OPERATION: AXILLOFEMORAL BYPASS (BILATERAL)

Position: Supine. Place the arm on the side to be used in the abducted position (Fig. 4-1).

Incision and Exposure: Make the femoral incisions first to determine the availability of the femoral arteries (Fig. 4-1). In conjunction with study of the arteriogram, this can be accomplished by external examination without opening the arteries.

Expose the axillary artery via an incision extending medially 8 cm. from the coracoid process 1 fingerbreadth below the clavicle (Figs. 4-1 and 4-2).

Separate the fibers of the pectoralis major.

Incise the costocoracoid membrane, sparing the anterior thoracic nerves if possible. Divide the pectoralis minor tendon at its origin on the coracoid process.

Divide the cephalic vein, which crosses the artery from lateral to medial.

Free up 4 cm. of the artery, dividing the superior thoracic artery if necessary.

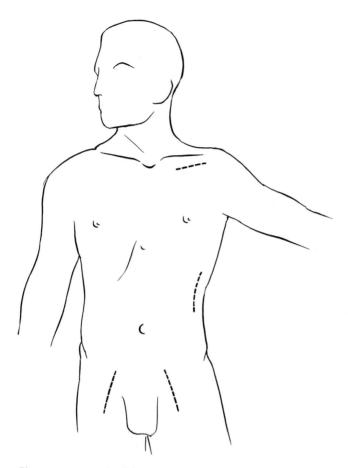

Figure 4-1.   Incisions.

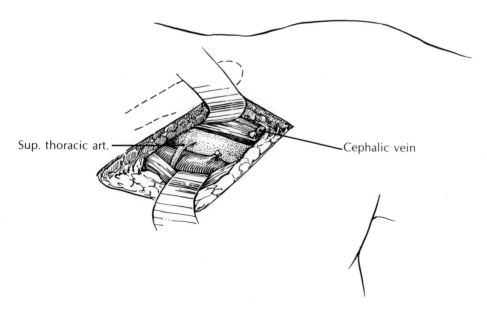

Sup. thoracic art.——————   ——Cephalic vein

Figure 4-2.   Exposure and dissection of axillary artery.

Subcutaneous Tunnels.   Make a tunnel subcutaneous to the ipsilateral common femoral (or external iliac) artery, using a tunneling instrument or a long clamp. Keep the tunnel in the midaxillary line until near the iliac crest. In most instances make an additional incision near the costal border to facilitate tunneling. Select the graft (10-mm. plastic prosthesis).

Make a suprapubic subcutaneous tunnel to the opposite common femoral or external iliac artery (see below). Select a suitable additional length of graft and suture it end to side to the first graft a few centimeters above the contemplated site of its lower anastomosis. Do not excise an ellipse of graft, as this reduces graft caliber.

Give 7500 units of heparin intravenously.

Draw the anteroinferior aspect of the axillary artery into the jaws of a curved vascular clamp so that a 3-cm. segment of artery will be maintained in a good position for suturing (Fig. 4-3).

Make a 17-mm. longitudinal arteriotomy. Arrange the tension and length of the main graft exactly so that the sidearm will later lie properly in its tunnel. Suture the prosthesis into the arteriotomy and test for leaks in the anastomosis by flushing with saline.

Place a right-angled clamp on the graft just distal to the anastomosis so that no blood can flow into the graft. Remove the vascular clamp to restore blood flow to the arm, and allow the axillary artery to fall back into its bed.

Draw the Y-graft down through the tunnel, taking care to avoid twisting. The orientation of the sidearm will help assure that it lies properly (Fig. 4-3).

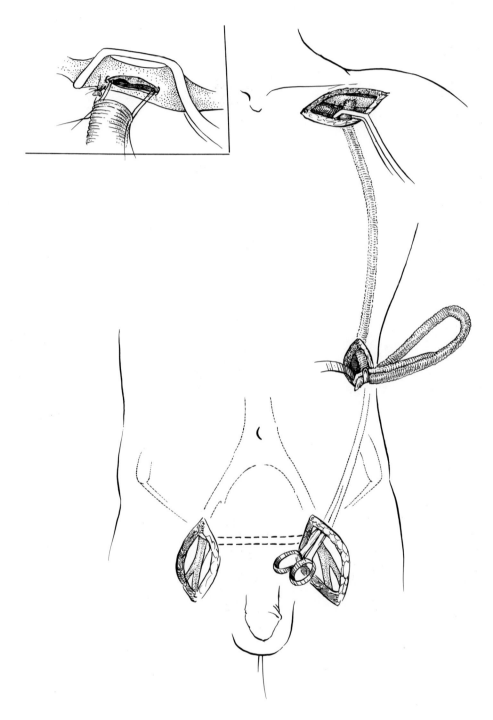

Figure 4-3.   Proximal anastomosis (*inset*), tunnel, and graft passage.

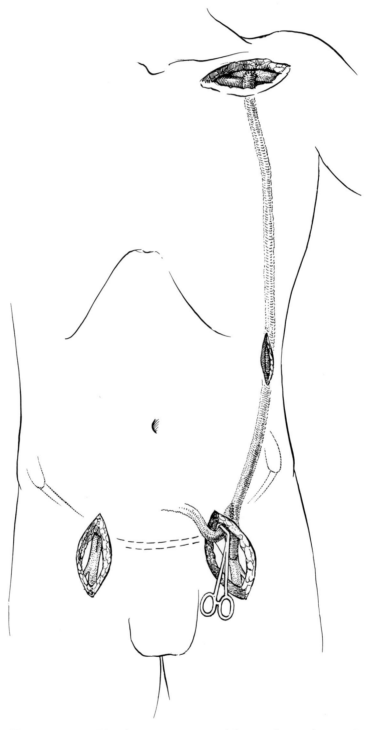

Figure 4-4.   Distal anastomosis and femorofemoral tunnel.

Trim the main graft to proper length at a 45-degree angle and suture the lower end to the ipsilateral common femoral artery. Test this anastomosis by flushing with saline through the sidearm.

Place a Kelly clamp on the sidearm next to its takeoff from the main graft (Fig. 4-4). Remove the femoral artery clamp and observe the graft for bleeding through its wall.

If bleeding is minimal, remove the upper clamp from the graft. Immediately substitute for this clamp the pinching action of the thumb and index finger of the left hand. Alternate bursts of high-pressure inflow lasting only 2 to 3 seconds with occlusion periods of 30 to 40 seconds until transmural graft bleeding has ceased.

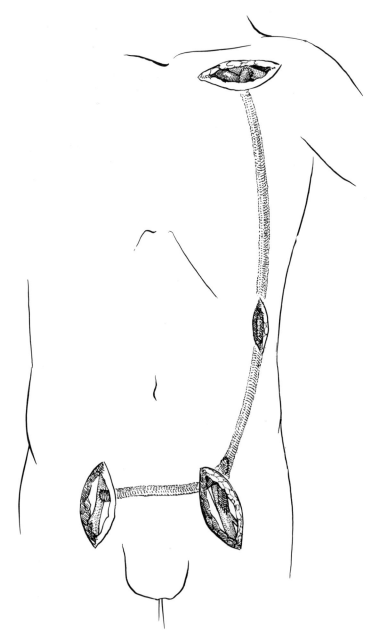

Figure 4-5.   Contralateral femoral graft anastomosis.

Draw the sidearm through its tunnel. Adjust it to the proper tension and trim the sidearm to length. Perform arteriotomy in the opposite common femoral artery suitably high and medially to receive the sidearm. Unite by end-to-side suture. Remove the clamps (Fig. 4-5).

Give 50 mg. of protamine sulfate slowly intravenously.

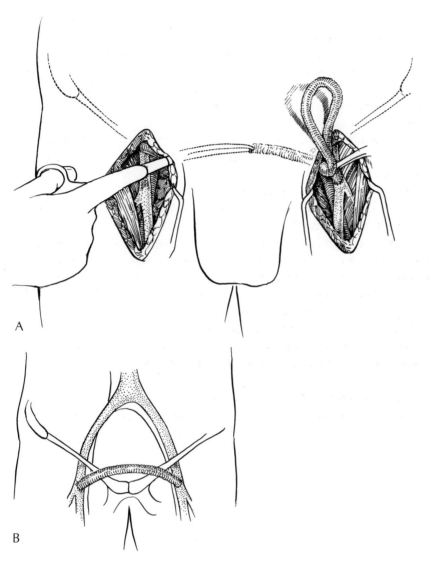

Figure 4-6.   (*A*) Femorofemoral graft, halfway done. (*B*) Femorofemoral graft, completed.

OPERATION: FEMOROFEMORAL BYPASS

Incision and Exposure: The same as for the lower incisions (Fig. 4-1).
  Expose the common femoral (or external iliac arteries) and assess them externally for caliber and quality.

Steps in Procedure: Make the suprapubic tunnel just anterior to the deep fascia.

Prepare the destinational common femoral artery as in Figures 3-6 or 3-7. Be sure that the arteriotomy is made high enough and medially enough so that the graft will lie without kinking as it emerges from the tunnel.

Perform only enough thromboendarterectomy to relieve obstruction of the common femoral or the deep femoral artery, or both. Otherwise, preserve the thickness of the wall provided by the arteriosclerotic process.

Perform the anastomosis of origin first and test this by flushing the preclotted graft with saline. Place a Kelly clamp on the graft next to its takeoff and restore flow to the good leg (Fig. 4-6A).

In performing the second anastomosis, it is important to suture the medial side first, and from above downward, so that the graft is free for accurate placement of each succeeding stitch.

When the operation has been completed (Fig. 4-6B), neither femoral artery should be lifted forward out of its bed, nor should the graft be redundant.

In both axillofemoral and femorofemoral grafting, several considerations help in deciding whether to use the external iliac artery just above the inguinal ligament in preference to the common femoral artery:

1. Adequate caliber of the external iliac artery.
2. Angiographic demonstration by oblique films that the mouth of the deep femoral artery is nonstenotic and that the common femoral is widely patent.
3. Prior operation on the common femoral.
4. The likelihood that subsequent femoropopliteal bypass may be done.

5 Femoropopliteal and femorotibial bypass for obliterative arteriosclerosis

FEMOROPOPLITEAL BYPASS

OBJECTIVE

To transport mainstream arterial flow beyond the block.

INDICATIONS

Rest pain, necrosis, or disabling intermittent claudication. Since later closure of the new channel is more common than in reconstructions for aortoiliac disease, indications for operation are more restricted. Whereas a degree of ischemia that threatens amputation is a firm indication for operation, we recommend it in patients with intermittent claudication only for disability that significantly interferes with the activities of daily living.

Arteriographic evidence of "localized" block. For femoropopliteal bypass the popliteal artery must be open for at least 2 cm. above its bifurcation, and the bifurcation must be visualized. Multiple or short blocks of the calf arteries do not contraindicate operation. If two calf arteries are closed, the third must be of good caliber and patency.

CONTRAINDICATIONS

Intermittent claudication that is not disabling.

No popliteal, tibial, or peroneal artery open below the block. While vein grafts sutured into "isolated popliteal segments" (collateral outflow only) have shown surprising patency rates, this pattern of obstruction calls for caution. If an unusually good tibial artery is present below the distal popliteal block, bypass to it should be considered.

PLANNING AND PREPARATION

Arteriography should be done. In diabetic patients, filming should be carried down to the ankle joint level.

Routine skin preparation.

Map the course of the saphenous vein with a skin marker the night before with the patient standing.

A two-team combination greatly expedites this procedure. One team dissects the arteries while the other removes and prepares the vein. The anastomoses are done simultaneously.

The preferred graft is the ipsilateral saphenous vein. If the lower anastomosis will be above the knee joint line, a knitted Dacron prosthesis is the second choice. If the lower anastomosis must lie below the knee joint line, a composite graft of vein and fabric is preferable.

The maintenance of vein graft patency with time correlates directly with the diameter of the vein. Venous segments less than 5 mm. in diameter should not be used. When the length of a vein of adequate caliber is insufficient to span the distance from the common femoral to the lower popliteal arteries, it is tempting to use the available vein as a limited bypass joining the lower femoral to the lower popliteal artery. Unless the upper segment of the femoral artery combines large caliber with a very smooth wall, this is a mistake. Obliterative arteriosclerosis progresses rapidly in the superficial femoral artery; it rarely obstructs the common femoral artery. A composite graft should be used in this situation.

The fourth choice for arterial replacement would be autologous cephalic vein. Thromboendarterectomy of the superficial femoral artery is undesirable because of fibrous reaction, narrowing, and gradual closure. Fibrin-digested bovine collagen grafts should not be used. An autologous connective tissue (mandril-prepared) graft represents an additional but still unsettled alternative, provided a six-week delay in function is feasible.

OPERATION

Position and Draping: Supine. Prepare the lower extremity from umbilicus to mid-foot, and drape it so that various positions of the leg from straight to frogged to 90 degrees can be assumed.

Incision and Exposure: The upper incision should be 6 cm. long and is made just medial to the femoral artery, which, whether pulsing or not, can be palpated in the femoral triangle. Extend the upper end of the incision to the inguinal ligament (Fig. 5-1). Try to come down directly on the saphenous vein by knife dissection so that the vein is completely exposed down to its adventitia. This permits much more accurate early appraisal of vein caliber,

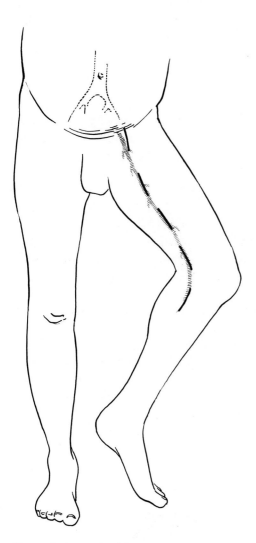

Figure 5-1.   Incision.

because venospasm due to tissue traction and vein wall stimulation is eliminated.

Dissection of Saphenous Vein: Continue the exposure of the saphenous vein, which runs obliquely and medially from its bulb of junction with the femoral vein. Perform finger dissection downward in the subcutaneous tissues between the vein and the skin and between the vein and the deep fascia. The branches will become evident. Divide them between clamps and ligate as you progress. Avoid undue traction, which will cause the branches to tear the vein wall and may injure the media of the vein itself. Ideal repair of a vein wall tear is virtually impossible.

Gentle tugging on the dissected vein will demonstrate precisely the course of the vein below. Make a second incision, 5 cm. long, over the vein at a point as far distal as possible from the first that will still allow further dissection from the point reached through the upper incision. Continue with further dissection and incisions until the proper length of vein is cleared. The supracondylar and infracondylar vein incisions are later used to approach the artery (Fig. 5-2). Take 5 to 6 cm. extra vein whenever possible.

The bifurcation of the saphenous vein in the thigh presents a challenge in that a decision must now be made as to which branch to continue dissecting. Choose the largest. If the branches are the same size, select the one that courses toward the saphenous cutaneous channel as marked on the skin 6 to 8 cm. medial to the patella. Occasionally the vein will divide into equal channels that reunite lower down, and such veins can be used intact. Leave the saphenous vein flowing in situ until the arterial dissections are completed.

Dissection of Femoral Artery: Dissect the femoral artery as in Figure 3-2 and identify the best site for arteriotomy by palpation over a right-angled clamp (see Fig. 2-2B), preferably low on the common femoral artery and somewhat medial. Do not perform arteriotomy at this time.

Dissection of Popliteal Artery: See Fig. 5-3.

If the popliteal artery below the block is patent and of good quality on arteriography for 5 cm. above the joint line, the skin incision can be made above the medial condyle and the site of lower anastomosis selected in the artery above the knee joint. If the cephalad end of satisfactory popliteal patency is below this, make the lower incision in the upper medial calf. Even though it is tempting to choose the upper incision to avoid placing the graft across the knee joint, it is unwise to dissect the popliteal artery at joint level or below through a supracondylar incision, since this will require the lower anastomosis to be done through a difficult exposure.

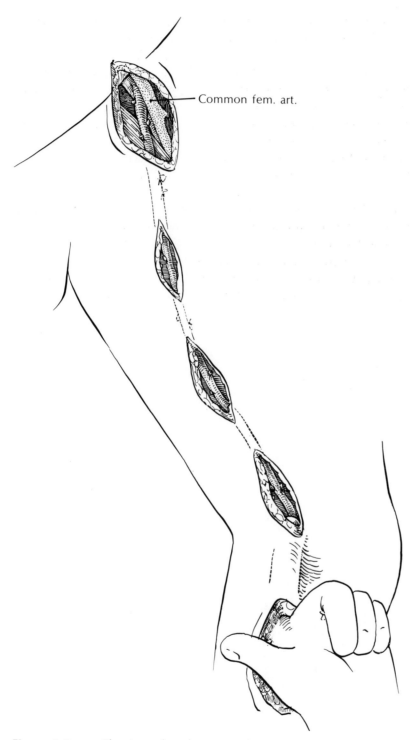

Common fem. art.

Figure 5-2.   Clearing of saphenous vein.

For the lower approach, "frog" the leg and deepen the incision by opening the deep fascia 1.5 cm. posterior to the easily palpable posterior edge of the tibia. This allows entry into the lower popliteal space. Palpate with the finger deep in the wound and identify the vascular bundle by rolling it against the posterior surface of the upper tibia; the tibial nerve is 1 to 2 cm. deep (lateral) to this. Although there is usually one principal popliteal vein, there are many uncharted branches and continuations of the sural venae comitantes that require dissection and ligation before the artery can be cleared. Dissect out 6 cm. of the artery to allow its elevation into the superficial area of the wound. Select the site of arteriotomy on the posteromedial surface of the artery.

The Tunnel: Dissection of the saphenous vein has already provided an appropriate tunnel at the subcutaneous level in the thigh. It is not necessary to carry the graft deep to the sartorius muscle. To dissect the lower end of the tunnel to the lower popliteal artery, approximate the forefingers of each hand, one in the popliteal space and one from above, between the adductor and hamstring tendons. The passage is through fatty and areolar tissue and is bloodless.

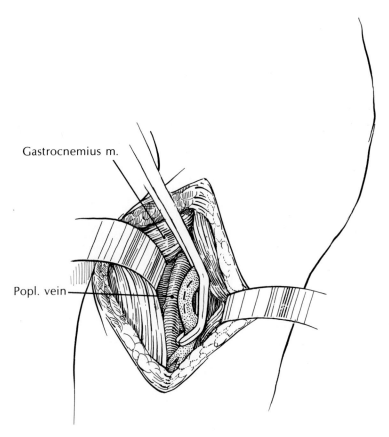

Gastrocnemius m.

Popl. vein

Figure 5-3.   Lower dissection (lower popliteal artery)—trial application of clamp.

Lower Anastomosis: Divide the saphenous vein graft at both ends, remove it, and test for leaks and constrictions, using blood obtained from the common femoral artery to which heparin has been added (Fig. 5-4). Avoid high syringe pressures, which can disrupt the venous media. Correct the leaks with 5-0 ligatures or sutures and the constrictions by dividing constricting bands with fine scissors. Give 7500 units of heparin intravenously. Place traction sutures of 4-0 monofilament close together on either side of the proposed arteriotomy. Using a right-angled clamp, lift the best segment of popliteal artery into a curved or Satinsky vascular clamp with the lock lying superiorly. Close the clamp very gently. Tent the arterial wall with traction sutures and make a single incision through all coats of the arterial wall into the lumen. Enlarge the incision with fine scissors to 10 to 15 mm. in length. Test for bleeding from both directions by removing and reapplying the temporary clamp.

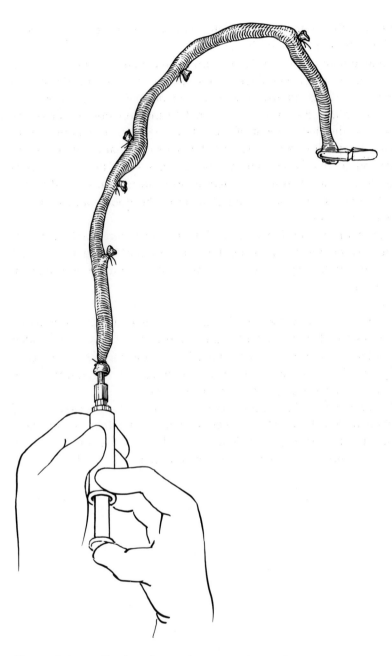

Figure 5-4.   Testing the saphenous vein graft.

After reversing the graft, resect the area crushed by the clamp. Remove adventitia from the cut end for about 2 cm.

Make a longitudinal incision of 12 mm. from the cut end. Suture the vein to the artery by the trumpet technique. Using a double-armed needle of 5-0 Tevdek (or two separate sutures as shown in Figure 5-5), make an everting mattress suture uniting the throat of the graft to the superior corner of the arteriotomy. Pass the first element of the suture over and over from vein to artery, the most difficult side first, down to the apex of the arteriotomy. Avoid drawing adventitial shreds through the suture holes since they create constricting bands of connective tissue. There is no need to trim more than the corners of the graft. Using the second element of the double-armed suture, sew the remaining side.

Test the anastomosis with Ringer's solution and close significant leaks with single sutures. By temporary removal of the clamp on the popliteal artery, test the ability to irrigate through the graft. Leave no blood in the tested segment after this maneuver.

Upper Anastomosis: Draw the graft through the tunnel, taking care to avoid rotation. Trim its length so that after the anastomosis it will lie without undue tension or redundancy. The error of cutting it too short cannot be compensated for by stretching, as can be done with a fabric graft. In adjusting graft length, be sure that the leg is extended at the knee.

Perform arteriotomy of the common femoral artery at the selected site and any thromboendarterectomy of the deep femoral artery that is indicated. Anastomose the vein graft to the arteriotomy. Gently dilate the vein just below the anastomosis with a right-angled clamp before putting in the last stitches.

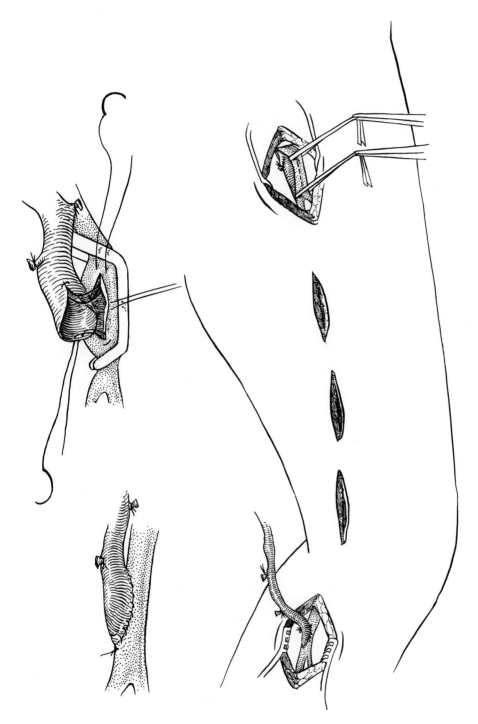

Figure 5-5.   Lower anastomosis, starting with two sutures completed, and relationship to graft tunnel.

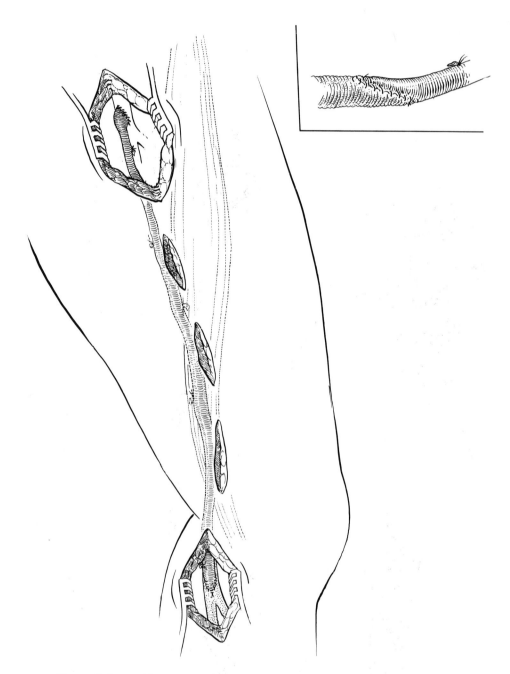

Figure 5-6.   Upper anastomosis completed. Composite graft (*inset*).

Remove the popliteal artery clamp first. Look for vein graft filling as proof of good backbleeding. Remove the femoral artery clamp. Search the tunnels for undue bleeding (Fig. 5-6).

Repair any leaks in the anastomosis or vein graft with the upper clamp briefly back in place. Suture hole leaks should be packed. Suture hole slits are closed with transverse adventitial 5-0 sutures. In the rare event that drainage is needed, place a Hemovac line in the tunnel. Remove it in 24 hours.

When a composite graft is selected (Fig. 5-6, inset), the central technical feature is creation of a long, smoothly tapering anastomosis at the graft-vein junction. This is easily accomplished when anastomosing a 6-mm. prosthetic graft to a 5-mm. vein. Most surgeons prefer an 8-mm. prosthesis, so the caliber discrepancy is far more striking. Cut the prosthesis very obliquely so that an oval opening 2 cm. in length will be created. Trim off the distal 2 to 3 mm. Open the throat of the prosthesis for another 5 mm. Cut the vein very obliquely to create an oval opening 2.5 cm. in length. Cut off the distal 2 to 3 mm. Open the throat of the vein for another 5 mm. The respective circumferences of the two approximately oval openings will be about the same. Suture the distal cut end of each graft to the throat of the other with a mattress suture that can be tied and then run along one side of the anastomosis and tied to its counterpart. Because the venous component of the anastomosis must be longer than that of the prosthesis, a slight angle will be formed at this junction. If the vein-to-prosthesis anastomosis is done before anastomosing the vein to the popliteal artery, the tunnel and the "lie" of the composite graft can be made to accommodate this angle.

FEMOROTIBIAL BYPASS

OBJECTIVE

To transport mainstream arterial flow from the femoral artery beyond the blocked popliteal into a tibial vessel.

INDICATIONS

Rest pain, necrosis, or disabling intermittent claudication.

The arteriogram must show a considerable segment of tibial or peroneal artery open from some level above the ankle continuously into one of the pedal arches. Injections of contrast material during reactive hyperemia may be helpful in showing the true patency of the distal arterial anatomy.

CONTRAINDICATIONS

Intermittent claudication that is not truly disabling (rare when the popliteal artery is closed).

An interrupted, narrow tibial vessel not joining a plantar arch.

VARIOUS SURGICAL APPROACHES

When the distal popliteal artery is thrombosed, the anterior and posterior tibial arteries at this bifurcation are almost invariably highly stenotic, with atheroma. The same is often true of the peroneal artery takeoff. Attempts to endarterectomize these segments involve difficult exposures, a high rate of venous injury, and very low success rates.

Surgical strategy rests on the angiographic identification below this trifurcation level of a clearly patent vessel of sufficient caliber and distal distribution, as just described. A variety of approaches are available (Fig. 5-7A).

For anastomoses to the proximal posterior tibial or peroneal arteries, use a medial incision just posterior to the tibia (Fig. 5-7B). This divides the tibial attachment of the soleus muscle, which is pushed posteriorly and reveals the posterior tibial artery just lateral to the posterior surface of the tibia. The peroneal artery is located in this same plane but further laterally as it enters the flexor hallucis longus muscle (Fig. 5-7C).

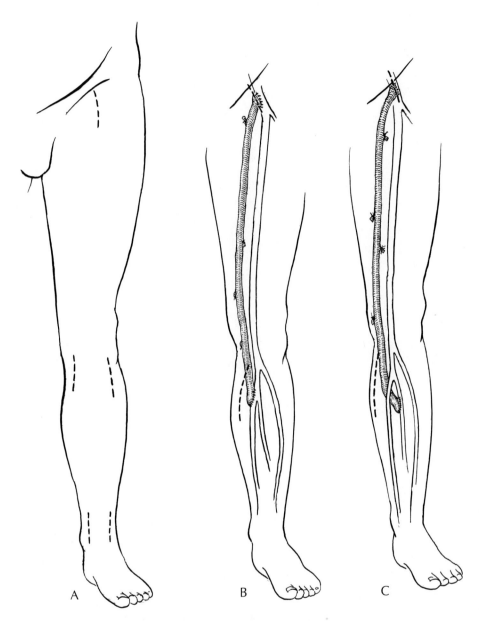

Figure 5-7.   (A) Femorotibial incisions. (B) Femoral-to-proximal posterior tibial bypass. (C) Femoroperoneal bypass.

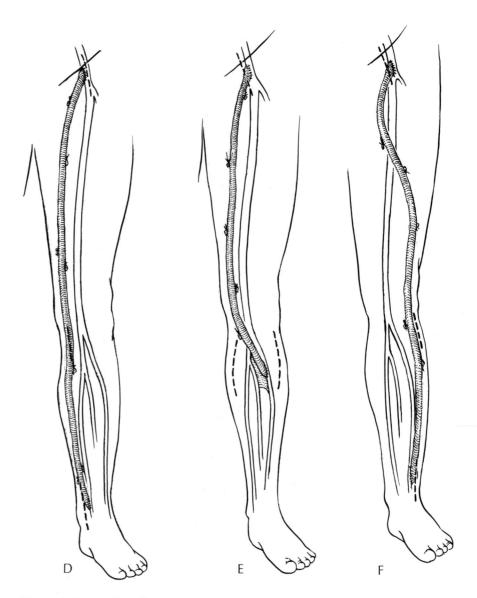

Figure 5-7 (continued).   (D) Femoral-to-distal posterior tibial bypass. (E) Femoral-to-proximal anterior tibial bypass. (F) Femoral-to-distal anterior tibial bypass.

Approach the anterior tibial artery through a vertical incision 2 cm. lateral to the tibial crest and just medial to the fibula, a route that passes through the lateral fibers of the anterior tibial muscle (Fig. 5-7E). The artery is found lying on the anterior surface of the interosseous membrane. Subperiosteal resection of the head of the fibula, which unroofs the popliteal bifurcation, is not necessary for these anterior tibial anastomoses.

The tunnel connecting either one of these exposures with the proposed site of graft takeoff (the common femoral artery is preferred) will follow the course of the popliteal artery. As described under femoropopliteal bypass, the medial supracondylar exposure of the upper popliteal artery is joined by blunt dissection along the course of the popliteal artery with either the anterior or posterior lower exposure. The tunnel runs deep to the sartorius muscle into the popliteal space between the heads of the gastrocnemius muscle. When joining this area to the anterior tibial exposure, the popliteal tunnel is opened along the anterior wall of that artery to continue along the anterior wall of the anterior tibial. Pierce the interosseous membrane just superior to the passage of the anterior tibial artery with the tip of a long, curved clamp in order to maintain this anterior relationship for passage of the vein graft and its anastomosis.

If the course of the popliteal artery has been used for a previous bypass graft, this tunnel cannot be easily created by blunt dissection. Either remove the old graft by careful exposure and full dissection or create a subcutaneous tunnel medial or lateral to the knee for the new graft.

For low anastomoses to the posterior (Fig. 5-7D) or anterior (Fig. 5-7F) tibial arteries, make vertical incisions directly over the corresponding artery just above the level of the malleoli. Proximal to this point the arteries lie deep in muscle, and distally they lie deep to many tendons.

For a posterior tibial procedure at the ankle, the graft tunnel is subcutaneous and medial all the way to the groin, following the course of the saphenous vein. In the case of an anterior tibial bypass, the graft tunnel is subcutaneous and lateral all the way up to the mid-thigh, which it crosses anteriorly to reach the common femoral artery.

OPERATION

The first choice of graft is the ipsilateral saphenous vein, and the first choice of graft takeoff is the common femoral artery. The superficial femoral artery is occasionally an excellent vessel of good caliber worthy of graft origin. Often the availability of satisfactory cephalic or basilic vein additions will determine the site at the graft takeoff.

Position and Draping: Routine skin preparation. Supine position. Prepare the lower extremity from umbilicus to mid-foot, and drape it so that various positions of the leg from straight to 90-degree flexion of the knee can be assumed. If saphenous vein quality and suitable length are in doubt, prepare one shoulder and the entire arm.

Exposure and Dissection: Expose and dissect the saphenous vein through multiple incisions to assess its caliber and useful length. Leave it in continuity (Fig. 5-2).

Dissect the distal artery of choice through one of the exposures previously described.

Isolate 3 cm. of distal artery, dividing and ligating small branches.

Dissect the proximal artery at the site of graft takeoff.

Bluntly dissect the graft tunnel as indicated.

Place small clamps or catgut loops on the distal artery after giving 7500 units of heparin intravenously. Make the distal arteriotomy first, using a small blade and then a Potts scissors, to a length of 8 to 10 mm. The artery may have to be held somewhat rolled over so that the anastomosis will permit smooth inflow from the graft at the proper angle. As in aortocoronary bypass grafts, use single rather than mattress sutures at the ends of the arteriotomy. Binocular loupes may be helpful.

Use 6-0 monofilament sutures for the lower anastomosis.

Gently dilate the artery proximally and distally with small dilators.

Removal and preparation of the saphenous vein, the anastomoses, care to avoid twisting in the tunnel, and avoidance of tension or kinks at suture lines are all as described for femoropopliteal bypass.

If composite grafts are used, end-to-end anastomoses cut very obliquely and hence made long (2.0 to 2.5 cm.) will satisfactorily smooth out disparities in caliber and wall thickness.

6 Complications of arterial reconstruction

INTRAOPERATIVE COMPLICATIONS

THROMBOSIS IN A RECONSTRUCTED SEGMENT

Example: Following aneurysm resection, removal of the final clamp from one iliac limb of the graft fails to restore the corresponding femoral pulse. Through a transverse incision in that limb of the graft, the Fogarty catheter recovers a good deal of clot from the external iliac artery; good backbleeding follows, even with the hypogastric artery clamped.

Here, insufficient heparin was used. Average-sized patients require 7500 units intravenously each hour. Backbleeding should have been assured before placing the last few sutures in the iliac anastomosis. Many surgeons routinely pass Fogarty catheters down each iliac artery prior to completing such anastomoses.

Example: If blood inadvertently enters a bypass graft while the second anastomosis is being done, the entire graft may fill with clot unless anticoagulation from heparin is complete. Under these circumstances, or after preclotting maneuvers, all gross clot must be milked, irrigated, or suctioned out of a graft.

ABNORMAL BLEEDING

Continuing diffuse bleeding resulting from clotting factor deficits, rather than from inadequate surgical hemostasis, is typically seen in patients with ruptured aneurysm who received many transfusions preoperatively and another 10 to 12 units of blood during the operation. Clots are not being formed anywhere in the field; irrigation with Ringer's solution reveals a steady ooze originating from innumerable minute vessels. Many clotting factors have been diluted out or consumed, particularly platelets.

Under these circumstances use tightly woven grafts and strictly avoid the loose knitted ones.

The first step in treatment is to give protamine sulfate to neutralize com-

pletely any residual heparin effect, which, with minimal renal excretion, may
be prolonged. Arrange for the administration of large amounts of fresh-frozen
plasma and several platelet transfusions as needed. Obtain urgent consultation with a hematologist and assay clotting factor deficiencies. The following
basic tests should be made:

1. Platelet count.
2. Fibrinogen concentration.
3. Euglobulin lysis time.
4. Fibrin split products.
5. Partial thromboplastin time.
6. Thrombin time.

Coagulation hemotologists vary in their diagnostic requirements and in-
terpretations.

When it is clear that additional suture ligatures or cautery coagulation of
bleeding points will not achieve hemostasis, suture the retroperitoneum over
Hemovac tubing brought out behind the left colon through the flank. Complete tissue coaptation is the best treatment for the oozing abdominal wound.

URETERAL INJURY

When aortoiliac reconstruction follows sigmoid or rectal resection, a failed
prior reconstruction, or retroperitoneal sepsis, the ureters may be densely
scarred and abnormally located. Thus, despite every precaution, including the
placement of ureteral catheters, inadvertent division of a ureter occasionally
occurs. It can be repaired as follows.

Free up the proximal and distal ureteral segments for 5 or 6 cm. so that the
site of repair will lie completely free of tension. Dilate each lumen gently with
a right-angled clamp. With sharp plastic scissors, cut back each end at a
45-degree angle to full-thickness normal ureter, avoiding any twist. Dilate
each lumen again. Using 5-0 chromic catgut through all layers, carry out
end-to-end anastomosis with nine or ten interrupted sutures. Use repeated
gentle dilatations of each lumen to ensure perfect visualization and placement
of each suture. Do not place a stint inside the ureter. Do not drain except for
a single Hemovac line placed next to the repair; remove this in 24 hours.

Separate the ureteral suture line from a vascular graft by a flap of retroperitoneal fat or by tacking down the retroperitoneum between the two.

A good ureteral anastomosis is completely watertight and heals very well.

An intravenous pyelogram in 48 hours will demonstrate a slender ureter
that is functioning well.

ATHEROTHROMBOTIC EMBOLISM

In operations for aneurysm or stenotic disease, when the aortoiliac arteries are found to be loaded with masses of old pale clot loosely adherent to atheromatous ulcers, it is easy to allow crumbs of intraluminal material to embolize distally during the operation.

This occurs in two settings. The first is when a tape that has been passed around the aorta or an iliac artery and used for traction to aid in dissection of that vessel angulates the artery and forces the axial stream of blood against one wall. The resulting strong jet effect can then blast embolic material downstream. The second follows a local endarterectomy, as of the abdominal aorta just below the renal arteries preparatory to aortofemoral bypass. Clots and atheromatous debris may be caught in either clamp, or lie above the upper clamp or below the lower one. Make every possible attempt to recover such loose material. Release the upper clamp briefly to flush debris down into the aortotomy site. Release the lower clamp briefly and extract debris back up out of the lower aorta by the careful use of a large bone curette.

POSTOPERATIVE COMPLICATIONS

RETROPERITONEAL AND INTRA-ABDOMINAL BLEEDING

Without any fault in the clotting mechanism, occasional patients will demonstrate a need for continuing blood replacement during the first 8 to 12 postoperative hours. This need is demonstrated by falling urine output, a drop in systolic blood pressure, an increase in measured abdominal girth, a lowering of the central venous pressure, and a positive response to transfusion. Serial hematocrit readings show a falling curve despite transfusions.

The decision to explore the operative site to control bleeding is obviously based on the rate of bleeding and its trend. While many factors influence the decision, the need for more than 5 or 6 units of blood during the first 8 to 12 hours usually dictates reoperation. Do not postpone the decision. The simple act of removing 3 to 4 liters of blood from the peritoneal cavity greatly improves respiratory exchange and hastens convalescence.

CLOSURE OF THE RECONSTRUCTION BY THROMBOSIS

During the afternoon of operation, or over the next few days, some arterial reconstructions will close.

When the reconstruction was done without great optimism in the presence of poor distal vessels in a patient with other severe disease, the decision may be not to reoperate. Under most circumstances, however, at least one thorough attempt should be made to restore blood flow through the reconstruction. Through transverse incisions in the graft or artery, use Fogarty catheters to clear out all obstructing thrombus. Hematomas of the tunnel, twisting or undue tension in a bypass, intimal flaps, sutures crossing the anastomosis, emboli from above, clamp injuries to intima, and inflow obstruction should all be considered as possible causes.

For example, if the Fogarty catheter will pass through the upper anastomosis of a common femoral-to-popliteal bypass vein graft only after considerable reduction in balloon size, that anastomosis should be revised. If the vein caliber is only 5 mm. and the anterior wall of the common femoral artery is very thick, a capacious, smooth-flowing anastomosis can be constructed using a venous patch. A vein patch 2.5 by 1.5 cm. is sutured to the common femoral arteriotomy, and the vein graft is anastomosed to a 1.5-cm. longitudinal venotomy in the patch. The width of the patch must be sufficient to provide enough vein to accommodate four suture lines.

Intraoperative arteriography after thrombectomy is most useful in pinpointing subtle defects.

Thrombectomy alone will rarely suffice; the cause of the thrombosis must be found and corrected if the new patency is to be maintained. The cause is often an unexpected one; each case should be approached with an open mind and the entire graft explored if necessary. Postoperative anticoagulation is not helpful.

ISCHEMIA OF THE SIGMOID COLON

After interruption of the inferior mesenteric artery in aneurysm resection or operations for aortoiliac stenosis, significant ischemia of the sigmoid occurs in 1 to 2% of cases. It is far more likely to occur when the inferior mesenteric and both hypogastric arteries are closed by disease, surgical division, embolic material, or intimal flaps. To maintain sigmoid blood flow, preserve both hypogastric arteries whenever reasonably possible. Check the sigmoid for color and arterial pulsations at the close of all these operations.

The first symptom of sigmoid ischemia is rectal bleeding. This evidence of acute mucosal ischemia may occur within a few hours of operation, but is more commonly seen a day or two later. Left lower quadrant pain is more worrisome; it suggests full-thickness injury. Diarrhea and tenesmus suggest muscle wall injury. Guarding and tenderness in the left lower quadrant in the wake of rectal bleeding and diarrhea (sometimes ileus) denote serosal involvement and dictate prompt exploration.

Under these circumstances, sigmoidoscopy is of little help because the depth of ischemic change cannot be estimated. Perform a low-level barium enema examination to look for "thumb-printing," air in the bowel wall, or barium in the bowel wall. Any of these findings would call for immediate exploration and sigmoid resection, usually with a temporary colostomy. Take great care not to open into the retroperitoneum over the graft.

COMPLICATIONS AFTER HOSPITAL DISCHARGE

SEPSIS

The most dreaded complication of arterial reconstruction is deep wound infection involving a prosthesis. Such infections stem from three different sources.

The first is a nidus of pathogenic bacteria (generally *Staphylococcus aureus*) residing in lymph channels or lymph nodes draining from a septic focus, usually in the foot. Dissection of the common femoral or popliteal arteries for bypass grafting can open into a septic lymphatic system and produce immediate bacterial contamination of the graft bed. Such septic foci in the limb should be drained and a four- to five-day course of bactericidal antibiotics used to sterilize the lymphatics prior to prosthetic grafting.

A second source, fortunately rare, is a septic focus, perhaps in the spine or lung, that feeds a septicemia. In this situation a suture line pocket containing thrombus can provide a target for secondary abscess and resulting suture line infection.

The most common type of wound sepsis involving an arterial reconstruction follows the intraoperative contamination of a clean field. Hematoma, the foreign-body effect of the prosthesis, and such contributing factors as extensive skin exposure, diabetes, and relative tissue or skin ischemia compound the danger from this cause. Adhesive plastic drapes covering bare skin areas should be used whenever feasible.

The most common site of wound sepsis from any cause is the region around the femoral artery, involving the lower end of an aortofemoral or upper end of a femoropopliteal bypass graft.

The classic evidences of femoral wound infection are fever, leukocytosis, local pain, tenderness, induration, and cellulitis. For an aortoiliac prosthesis, however, until the first suture line hemorrhage occurs, the only manifestations of infection are unexplained fever, night sweats, and leukocytosis.

Management of Sepsis Adjacent to a Prosthesis: Early detection and prompt drainage of infection overlying a prosthesis is the best hope for its salvage.

Such infections will often lie superficial to the deep fascia, so that open drainage of the skin and fat may be curative.

Deep infections involving a prosthetic suture line always lead to hemorrhage. The first hemorrhage is often small; recurrence is invariable. A suture line hemorrhage occurring more than a day or two but less than six months after operation almost always means a septic suture line. It calls for urgent removal of the prosthesis, debridement of the arteriotomy, and closure of the vessel with monofilament suture.

If a graft has thrombosed and sepsis involves its tract, the entire graft must be removed.

When a graft is still patent and the suture line has not bled, an attempt should be made to save the graft. Expose the infected area completely. Confirm the diagnosis by a direct smear with gram stain. Make cultures. Debride and curette the infected tract as thoroughly as possible. Lay a fine irrigating catheter with multiple perforations along the graft for instillations of antibiotic solution. Place a drain or suction sump at the far end of the system to remove excess irrigant. Use a suitable muscle flap, such as the sartorius of vastus medialis in the thigh, to cover the graft and suture line and eliminate dead space. Close the deep fascia. Leave the skin and subcutaneous tissue open. Suitable antibiotics are used intravenously at high dose levels.

Whenever infection is demonstrated at one end of a graft, it is important to know how far along the wall the process has spread. The number of days that fever has been observed, the amount of gross purulent exudate encountered, and the looseness of the graft in its fibrous tissue capsule are helpful clues to the extent of involvement. A "sinogram" made by injecting radiopaque dye through a small catheter in the tract of the graft can be very helpful.

If sepsis is limited to one end of the graft, approach the other end through a clean field and doubly ligate and divide the graft. The clean end of the graft tunnel is closed with one or two catgut sutures. Smears confirm the absence of bacteria in the clean field. Remove the remaining segment of "clean graft" unless, of course, it is functioning, as in one limb of an aortofemoral bypass.

Replace a septic aortoiliac prosthesis with an axillofemoral graft. If the common femoral artery must be sutured shut, so that deep femoral artery flow is lost when removing an infected prosthesis, consider an obturator canal bypass.

FALSE ANEURYSM

The development of a false aneurysm at a graft-host artery junction occurs most commonly at the femoral end of an aortofemoral bypass; the femoral end of a femoropopliteal bypass is the next most common site; the aortic end of an aortic prosthesis is probably third. Those developing in the first six weeks after operation can be caused by either infection or a minute, continuing leak. Those appearing between six weeks and six months are almost all caused by sepsis. Those appearing after six months (up to 10 to 12 years) are due to infraction of the silk suture material or gradual disruption of the arterial wall. Disruption is more frequent when a graft is sutured to an endarterectomized segment.

The diagnosis of false aneurysm at the femoral level is clearly based on demonstration of an expansile pulsation in an enlarging mass. At the aortic level, diagnosis is most difficult. Severe, constant back pain from bone erosion at the L2 to L3 level is the only complaint. In thin patients, demonstrable widening of the aortic pulsation on physical examination may be detectable. Aortography or an echo scan may confirm the diagnosis.

Since aneurysms all ultimately rupture, surgical treatment is imperative. The key decision in each case rests on the possibility of sepsis. This issue must be decided on the basis of the time relationships previously mentioned and direct smears made from the sac wall and the suture line.

Procedure: Control the arterial channels above and below the aneurysm.
    Dissect out the sac as far as possible.

Because of the thin-walled, fibrous nature of the sac, it is usually entered during attempted dissection. At times, the connection between the sac and the suture line is only a pinhole; occasionally the prosthetic graft is partly or wholly separated from the host artery at the suture line, and only the fibrous sac joins the two lumens.

When the anastomotic leak feeding the aneurysm is just a pinhole, a single two-bite suture will often solve the problem. When the false sac surrounds a large suture line dehiscence at the common femoral end of a bypass graft, it is several years after operation, and the smears are negative for bacteria, trim away the sac and curette the rim of compressed fibrin from the end of the graft and from the intimal side of the arteriotomy. Carefully pick out all old suture material, using a mosquito hemostat and a small blade. Frequently, the end of the graft can be neatly trimmed and the anastomosis done over, taking larger, deeper bites of artery and graft with monofilament sutures.

At times, the graft will be too short after trimming, and a short segment of new graft must be added.

If the arteriotomy edge is soft and friable and smears are positive, the graft must be removed; debride the arteriotomy and nearby tissues and close the arteriotomy.

Procedure in Aortic False Aneurysm: When the false aneurysm is at the upper anastomosis of an abdominal aortic graft, do not endeavor to gain proximal control by circumferential dissection of the aorta at any point, and do not attempt to dissect the false aneurysm initially.

Identify the old graft at its midportion and bluntly dissect away the surrounding fibrous capsule circumferentially. A large pulmonary lobe forceps firmly grasping a rolled-up gauze sponge is held in position on the aorta just above the superior mesenteric artery for instant compression if needed. Cautiously dissect the graft almost up to its junction with the false aneurysm.

Ensure high urine output with an intravenous water load, furosemide (Lasix), or mannitol if necessary.

Doubly clamp the graft and make a transverse incision between the clamps through the anterior half of the graft. Introduce a Foley catheter with a 30-cc. bag into the graft. With the aorta occluded by compression above, remove the upper clamp and pass the bag through the graft lumen to a position just above the false aneurysm. Inflate the balloon snugly against the aortic wall. This will usually occlude both renal artery ostia. The strong force of the aortic pulse will tend to extrude the slippery balloon. Keep the aortic compressor in the ready position (Fig. 6-1B).

Now open the false aneurysm. Cut the aortic stump and the end of the graft free with the scissors and pick out the old suture material lying in the graft. The graft and aorta are usually easily reapproximated. Using 3-0 monofilament Dacron, and taking large bites of graft and aorta, put the posterior suture line in from within the lumen, inverting the cuff into the lumen toward the operator. This does not cause thrombosis or interfere with blood flow, and it makes the posterior half of the suturing far easier than attempting the conventional everting suture. The first suture starts at the midpoint of the back row and is carried 90 degrees toward the patient's right. Start the second suture so that it will just overlap the first, and carry it 90 degrees toward the patient's left. At this point, bring it outside the aorta, carry it over and over from left to right as an everting anterior suture line, and tie it to the first stitch. Make the transition from inversion to eversion of the suture line at each lateral aspect gradually over three to four bites of the suture.

The goal is to reunite the old graft and the host aorta in 20 to 25 minutes, so that the Foley catheter can be removed and renal blood flow restored before renal tubular injury results. If a new graft is needed, the suture line is placed as in Chapter 1, except that large bites and a single suture line are used in the interest of time.

Reapply aortic compression, remove the balloon, and reapply the original clamp above the opening in the graft, which is then closed (Fig. 6-1C).

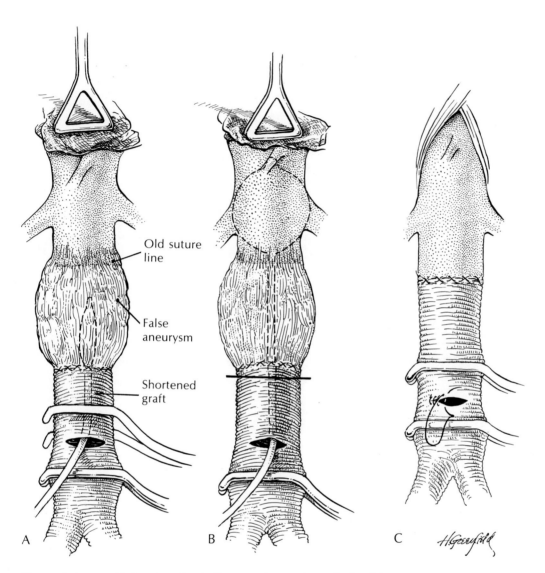

Old suture
line

False
aneurysm

Shortened
graft

A   B   C

Figure 6-1.   (A) Passing the balloon catheter through the false aneurysm.
(B) Proximal control obtained. (C) Completing the repair.

LATE THROMBOSIS

In femoropopliteal bypass grafts it is sometimes possible to detect a gradual falloff in pulsatile fllow by oscillometry or pressure recording, using ultrasound detection of flow during follow-up examinations. Arteriography can demonstrate a developing, well-localized stenosis, which can be treated by a relatively minor procedure prior to graft closure.

Far more common is the apparently sudden, complete closure that leads to return of the symptoms that prompted reconstruction. When collateral flow is good, late thrombosis occasionally may go undetected by the patient.

The decision for reoperation will depend on the extent of new ischemia, severity of the symptoms, estimated likelihood of success, the patient's fitness, and his acceptance. When one limb of a bilateral aortofemoral bypass graft closes, reoperation is indicated. Flow can sometimes be restored through an operation limited to the groin. Otherwise, replace the closed iliac limb by a new graft, using an oblique extraperitoneal approach to the graft's bifurcation (see Figs. 8-1 and 8-2).

The fault in these closures is usually found in a circumferential mass of compressed fibrin that lines both the graft and the common femoral artery at the anastomosis. If the graft is cut across 2 cm. above the anastomosis, this material can be curetted out and the inside of the anastomosis inspected without dissecting out the three arteries concerned. If backbleeding is not impressive, Fogarty catheters should be passed, and an arteriogram should be considered. If the anastomosis looks satisfactory, it need not be taken down. In this case, anastomose the iliac graft segment to this short segment of the original graft. Avoid tension on the anastomosis, which will increase with hyperextension of the thigh, and leave the deep fascia loose about the graft.

In attempting to declot any thrombosed fabric graft by Fogarty catheter manipulation, two problems commonly arise. The first results from circumferential fracture of the soft pseudointima when anything but very gentle crossclamping is used to control flow through such a graft. The second follows dislodgment of a cylindrical cast of this pseudointima as the result of traction of the inflated balloon. Either of these events guarantees recurrence of thrombosis.

Gain early control of the proximal end of the thrombosed graft segment to prevent undue blood loss during graft instrumentation. Scrape the entire prosthesis completely clean of any acquired lining using common bile duct scoops and bone curettes. Any shreds left behind can cause recurrence of thrombosis.

7 Arterial embolectomy

OBJECTIVE

To restore mainstream arterial flow to the limb before irreversible ischemic damage or distal thrombosis occurs.

INDICATIONS

Embolism to a major artery.

Emboli that can be removed easily under local anesthesia (brachial, femoral) should always be operated on even though survival of the limb seems likely otherwise.

CONTRAINDICATIONS

Late embolism (over 24 hours), when the fate of the limb is settled (gangrene or survival definitely established), is a contraindication to emergency operation. But "lateness" is not a contraindication to embolectomy if the fate of the limb still hangs in the balance. Moreover, elective late embolectomy after arteriography can be done successfully days or even weeks after embolism lodgment. After several days, these clots become adherent to the intima and must be approached directly rather than retrieved by catheter manipulation.

PLANNING AND PREPARATION (LOWER EXTREMITY EMBOLISM)

Identify the site of the embolus first by finding the level of the lowest palpable pulse. If this is at the femoral triangle, place an oscillometer or blood pressure cuff on the thigh above the femoral condyle. If this demonstrates a significant oscillation, it means that the superficial femoral artery is open and that a large embolus has lodged in the popliteal artery.

It is also true that a small popliteal embolism may obstruct the whole trifurcation and yet for a time allow palpation of the pulse above it in the popliteal space. In thin patients, the "thrusting" nature of the arterial pulsation above the site of embolism can at times be demonstrated. Because of variations in collateral circulation, the "level of demarcation," if present, is

Figure 7-1.   Arteriographic patterns of embolism (*left*) and thrombosis (*right*).

of no help in detecting the level of embolism. In popliteal embolism the calf oscillations are nearly or completely abolished.

Perform arteriography under the following circumstances: (1) when the level of embolism is in doubt (rare); (2) when the diagnosis (as opposed to thrombosis) is in doubt; and (3) when operation is not urgent (as in late embolism). The arteriographic pattern of embolism is different from that of thrombosis (Fig. 7-1).

To illustrate: A 30-year-old woman with mitral stenosis and atrial fibrillation has suffered previous embolic episodes. She presents with a 3-hour history of pain, coldness, and paralysis in her right foot. The lowest palpable pulse is the femoral. There is no oscillation in the thigh. In this case, do not do preoperative arteriography. For one year, a 70-year-old man with arteriosclerotic heart disease and atrial fibrillation has had some fatigue of the legs on walking. He presents with a 3-hour history of pain, coldness, and paralysis in the foot. The lowest palpable pulse is in the femoral artery. In this case, perform arteriography.

When emboli cause disappearance of the femoral pulse, prepare the whole abdomen as well as the involved leg(s) to the ankle.

Heparin (5000 units) is given intravenously as soon as the diagnosis of arterial occlusion is made. Heparinization is continued until circulation is restored.

OPERATION

Position: Supine.

Incisions: See Figure 7-2.

For aortic bifurcation ("saddle") embolism make incisions at both femoral sites. For femoral embolism make the same type of femoral incision on the indicated side. For fresh popliteal embolism work through a similar femoral incision. For embolism several days to weeks old use a medial incision below the knee joint, entering the popliteal space as on page 58.

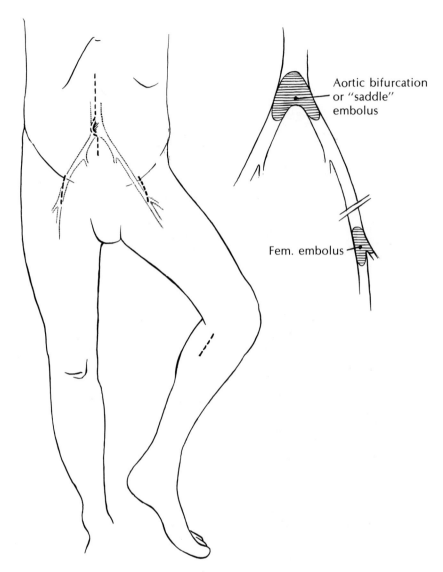

Figure 7-2.   Incisions and diagram for aortic bifurcation embolism and femoral embolism.

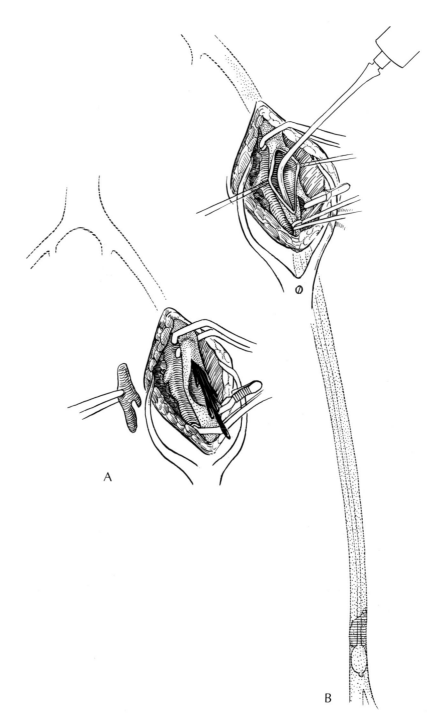

Figure 7-3.   (*A*) Femoral embolectomy. (*B*) Popliteal embolectomy using Fogarty catheter.

Details of Procedure: In aortic bifurcation or femoral embolism, dissect the origins of the superficial femoral and deep femoral arteries first, and apply bulldog clamps before disturbing the common femoral artery.

For unilateral iliac bifurcation embolism, shown by arteriogram, only the ipsilateral femoral artery need be controlled.

Dissect the common femoral artery (except in the direct popliteal approach) and perform a 3-cm. arteriotomy. Arteriotomy in the small-caliber superficial femoral artery should be avoided if possible. If it must be done there, it should be made transversely so that its closure will not constrict the lumen.

Remove the embolus locally (Fig. 7-3A) or from above with or without the help of a Fogarty catheter; to remove an embolus from below the femoral arteriotomy always use a catheter (Fig. 7-3B), making two or three additional passes after retrieving the last clot. Inject heparinized Ringer's solution via the irrigating catheter into the artery after the first catheter passes. Even though the patient is usually heparinized, these irrigations sometimes loosen additional clots.

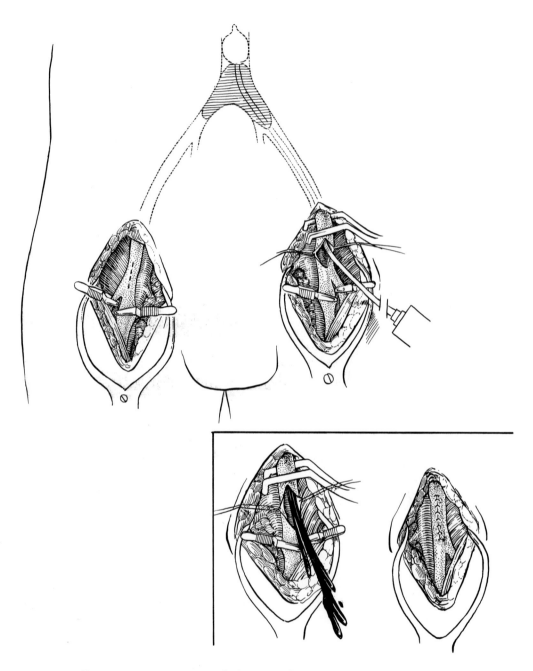

Figure 7-4.   Aortic embolectomy from below.

In an embolus above the femoral region involving one iliac artery, the catheter is used from the outset. After embolectomy insist on strong arterial flow from above. The spurt of free blood should project beyond the patient's foot (Fig. 7-4, *inset*). If the embolus involves the aortic bifurcation, control the superficial femoral and deep femoral arteries bilaterally and extract clot with the catheter first from one side and then from the other (before closing the arteriotomy in the first side) (Fig. 7-4).

In either aortic or unilateral iliac embolism, if strong arterial flow is not obtained, consider a direct approach to the aortic or iliac bifurcation to remove old embolus or previously unsuspected arteriosclerotic plaques. An alternative in a high-risk patient is a femorofemoral or axillofemoral graft (Chapter 5).

Since lesser emboli are lodged below large-vessel emboli in 25% of cases, an invariable rule of embolectomy is to make several passes of the catheter downward.

The intra-arterial injection of contrast material may be made either through the open arteriotomy or through a No. 18 needle after closure of the arteriotomy. In either case, it is well to clamp the artery above the injection site temporarily. If pedal pulses do not return after closing the arteriotomy, repeat the arteriography.

Continue systemic heparinization throughout the operative procedure.

POSTOPERATIVE MANAGEMENT

Heparin, while not necessary for prevention of local thrombosis after a successful embolectomy resulting in restoration of distal pulses, should be used to prevent recurrent embolism in all cases except those in which the operation wound contraindicates it. Practically speaking, this means all except abdominal wounds, and in such wounds start heparin after 24 hours.

Early operation on the mitral valve should be considered in patients with mitral stenosis. Use long-term anticoagulation in all such patients.

NOTE ON UPPER EXTREMITY EMBOLISM

In axillary and brachial artery embolism, the site of incision will depend on the level of pulse loss. If arterial pulsation is absent in the axilla, approach the brachial artery at the midhumeral level. It is easy to extract an embolus with the Fogarty catheter from below the level of lodgment.

If the brachial artery pulsation is felt almost down to the elbow, make the incision at the insertion of the biceps tendon so that the radial and ulnar artery origins can be dissected out and each vessel separately explored with the Fogarty catheter after removal of the embolus at the main bifurcation.

8 Thrombectomy and/or repair for acute arterial thrombosis of the lower extremity

ILIAC OR FEMOROPOPLITEAL THROMBOSIS

OBJECTIVE

To restore mainstream arterial flow before irreversible tissue damage occurs.

INDICATIONS

Gradual or sudden thrombosis is the final stage of all arterial stenotic processes, some of which are discussed in Chapters 2 through 5. This chapter deals only with sudden thromboses that create ischemia so massive as to require immediate attention.

A short (4-hour maximum from onset) period of observation under heparin (5000 units given immediately on diagnosis) is required to determine whether or not the collateral circulation is adequate to maintain viability long enough to allow an elective repair. Signs of nonviability (provided improved perfusion is not obtained) are the following:

Persistent loss of sensation in the toes.

Persistent painful rigor of the calf musculature. Loss of power of movement of the toes or ankle indicates more massive ischemia than the above, and, unless failure of movement is caused by pain, is a confirmatory indication.

Other indications are striking coldness, marked pallor or duskiness, and a very slow "pinking" time of the digits.

CONTRAINDICATIONS

None, other than intercurrent disease that renders the patient moribund.

PLANNING AND PREPARATION

Determine the level of occlusion, as in Chapter 7.

Even though the level may seem clear on examination, preoperative arteriography is indicated in most instances of thrombosis. The only exception is early postoperative thrombosis of an arterial reconstruction, where the site and nature of the arterial wall are known. For successful lasting restoration of circulation in a diseased artery, it is not enough to remove the thrombus. The lesion that caused it must also be removed (thromboendarterectomy) or bypassed. Arteriography will at least reveal the condition of the artery proximal to the occlusion and at most might show the patency of distal channels so that the extent of arterial reconstruction can be planned.

For thromboses above the inguinal ligament, prepare for axillofemoral, femorofemoral, or iliofemoral bypass. For a lesion below the inguinal ligament, prepare for common femoral thromboendarterectomy or, if it is distal to the femoral bifurcation, femoropopliteal or femorotibial bypass.

If the occlusion is at the femoral bifurcation or higher, the focus for distal runoff after reconstruction is the deep femoral artery. Restoration of flow to this artery by thrombectomy and thromboendarterectomy above it, or by bypass to it, will usually salvage the limb, even though the superficial femoral artery below it remains blocked.

When thrombosis in the superficial femoral and popliteal arteries is so extensive as to cause massive ischemia, the problem is more difficult. This is because the pattern of arterial stenosis that leads to popliteal thrombosis is much more extensive than that seen in the simple claudicator. In addition to the well-tolerated prior closure of the superficial femoral artery in the adductor canal, the popliteal artery itself has thrombosed because marked narrowing of the tibial and peroneal arteries has resulted in high resistance and poor flow. Thus a femoropopliteal bypass done to such a thrombectomized popliteal artery will usually thrombose for the same reason that the popliteal artery did. Under these circumstances, the best hope may lie in the possibility that one of the tibial arteries is highly stenotic at its ostium but of good caliber below this level, so that a femorotibial bypass is feasible.

Because of sluggish collateral circulation, the patency of one of the calf arteries that is so necessary to this procedure may be difficult to establish by preoperative arteriography. Intraoperative arteriography is done by hand injection into the common femoral artery below an occlusive clamp after thrombectomy by Fogarty catheter. As the catheter has to pass through a stenosis in the adductor canal, thrombectomy and the angiograms that follow it are often less than satisfactory. In this case, the next step will be arteriography via a cleared popliteal artery.

OPERATION

Position: Supine.

Incision: Make the incision in the femoral region as shown in the lower portions of Figures 3-1 and 3-2.

Procedure: If the lower end of the thrombosis is at the femoral bifurcation, perform femoral thromboendarterectomy (Fig. 3-6). If thrombosis is above this level, open the femoral artery and remove as much thrombus from below as possible using the Fogarty catheter. Unless retrograde intraoperative arteriography then shows no arterial disease, perform femorofemoral, axillofemoral, or iliofemoral bypass (see special note on iliofemoral bypass, p. 92).

If the thrombosis is distal to the femoral bifurcation, perform thrombectomy using the Fogarty catheter and intraoperative arteriography to ascertain the existence of an adequate popliteal or tibial artery branch for bypass. If one is found, perform bypass using a saphenous vein (see Chap. 5).

As mentioned, thrombectomy may not be complete enough to permit good visualization of the tibial vessels. If so, expose the popliteal artery and dissect out the upper 1.5 cm. of the anterior and posterior tibial arteries; open the popliteal in such a way that the incision can be extended into either of these vessels. Favor the larger artery. With stay sutures in the popliteal arteriotomy and no clamps applied, remove all thrombus; watch closely for any backbleeding from either the anterior or posterior tibial arteries. Inspect the ostium of each vessel directly for stenosis. Gently insert the tip of a right-angled clamp to calibrate the size of the ostium. Dilate both ostia if possible. This may produce much-increased backbleeding. Pass the Fogarty catheter down each artery, not only to extract any possible clot but also to map out obstructions and demonstrate changes in caliber. Ideally, one is looking for the situation that will permit the balloon catheter to pass to the foot, to be withdrawn smoothly at the 4 to 5 mm. caliber, but to check sharply at the takeoff of the tibial vessel.

Extend the arteriotomy through the ostium of this artery and make separate arteriograms of the anterior and posterior tibial arteries. If one good artery is found, the lower anastomosis of the saphenous vein bypass can be used to widen out the takeoff of this vessel.

If both arteries are irregularly and markedly narrowed, the catheter obstructs at numerous points, and backbleeding is negligible, no reconstruction can be done; the popliteal artery and operative incision are closed.

POSTOPERATIVE CARE

Heparinization, begun before the operation and continued throughout, should not be continued postoperatively. Otherwise, the routine is similar to that described for the type of reconstruction used.

ILIOFEMORAL BYPASS FOR ILIAC ARTERIAL THROMBOSIS

PLANNING AND PREPARATION

Arteriography performed via the contralateral femoral artery will show the level of occlusion of either the common iliac or external iliac artery. Most often the occlusion will involve the common iliac artery 1 cm. or so below the aortic bifurcation. Arteriography may show sufficient stenosis of the opposite iliac artery to contraindicate a femorofemoral bypass.

A unilateral extraperitoneal operation is generally well tolerated. The postoperative course is characterized by less incisional pain, less inhibition of pulmonary and gastrointestinal tract function, and better wound healing than is seen after full-scale abdominal aortic procedures.

OPERATION

Position: Supine.

Incision and Exposure: See Figure 8-1.

If the arteriogram has not shown clear refilling of the common and deep femoral arteries—and often it will not—a 7-cm. skin incision is made directly over the bifurcation of the common femoral artery from a point 1 cm. below the inguinal ligament. The common femoral artery, together with the proximal 1.5 cm. of the superficial femoral and deep branches, is freed up and carefully palpated for patency and major stenoses. The common femoral artery will usually be open. Occasionally, fresh thrombus can be removed from it and backbleeding obtained from the deep femoral artery ostium. Rarely the common femoral artery will be thrombosed, as will the proximal 2 cm. of the deep femoral artery. Endarterectomy of the deep femoral artery ostium may restore backbleeding in this vessel. The purpose of this initial exploration of the common and deep femoral arteries, as in the aortofemoral bypass, is to be sure at the outset that iliac reconstruction is possible.

After this common femoral dissection—which is omitted if the arteriogram shows refilling of the distal external iliac and common femoral arteries—make

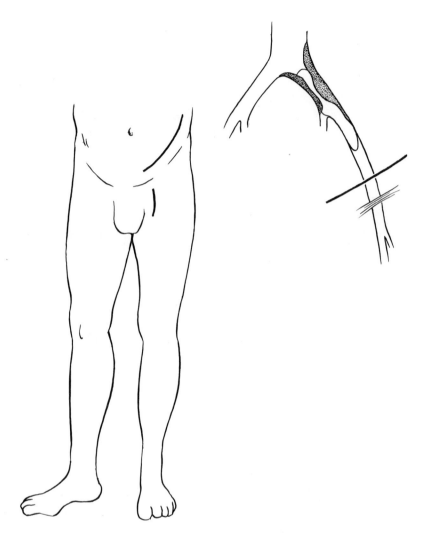

Figure 8-1.   Incisions for iliofemoral bypass and diagram of the thrombosis.

an oblique incision from just above the pubic tubercle, parallel to and 1 cm. above the inguinal ligament and curving superiorly just medial to the anterior superior spine of the ileum (Fig. 8-1). If both incisions are needed, preserve a 2-cm. skin bridge over the inguinal ligament. Deepen the incision through the aponeurosis of the external oblique muscle and split the fibers of this muscle laterally. Cut the internal oblique muscle directly across with shallow sweeps of the knife in the line of the skin incision. Open the fascia transversalis parallel to the inguinal ligament and 1 cm. above it, taking care not to open the underlying peritoneum.

Dissection of Iliac Artery: The pulseless external iliac artery is readily felt through the properitoneal fat and areolar tissue, usually as a beaded cord. The anterior wall is easily cleared by blunt dissection, sweeping the peritoneum upward and medially. Place a moist gauze pad over the superior margin of the incision and over the fold of peritoneum. Place the tip of a 2-inch Deaver retractor of suitable depth directly on the front wall of the artery. Sharp and blunt dissection, together with increasing traction and frequent repositioning of this retractor, will gradually clear the iliac arteries up to the aorta. The ureter, which crosses the iliac artery bifurcation, will adhere to the peritoneum and be lifted up with it.

When the iliac bifurcation is exposed, dissect the distal common iliac free from the underlying vein and encircle it with a tape. Frequent repositioning of the Deaver retractor and sharp and blunt freeing of the iliac artery will bring the operator to a strong pulse, either of the common iliac stump or of the aorta itself. Only enough of the aortic bifurcation to permit application of a clamp above all the thrombus need be freed up. Do not occlude or injure the intima of the opposite common iliac artery.

If the arteriogram has shown a common femoral of good caliber and an external iliac small in caliber or containing many plaques, make no effort to dissect the vessel circumferentially but decide on a bypass graft immediately and use 8- or 10-mm. Dacron, depending on the caliber of the host vessels. Consider thromboendarterectomy only for rare short obstructions of the common or external iliac with good quality artery above and below. Much time is wasted when an attempted endarterectomy ends up as a grafting procedure.

Give 7500 units of heparin intravenously.

If the common iliac artery is closed, it is easiest to transect this vessel 1.5 cm. below the upper clamp. Curette out any residual thrombus with a medium bone curette and carry out end-to-end anastomosis (Fig. 8-2). Flush out this segment to be sure that no clot or occluding atheroma remains above the anastomosis. Simultaneously test the anastomosis for leaks. Irrigate the blood out of the graft. It is worth emphasizing again that the common iliac

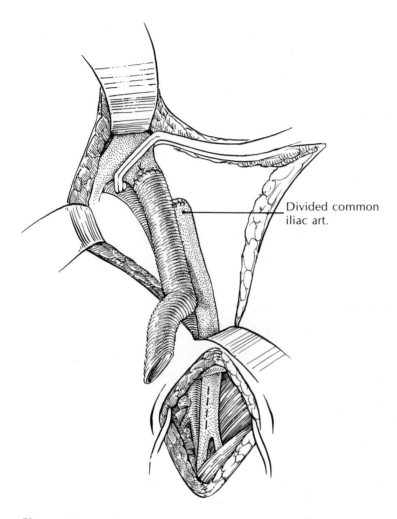

Divided common
iliac art.

Figure 8-2.   Upper anastomosis. Dacron graft to common iliac artery
stump, end-to-end.

takeoff or the aortic bifurcation itself must be freed up enough so that the
upper clamp is placed on a thin-walled, strongly pulsatile artery.

If the primary iliac stenosis is at the iliac bifurcation or in the external iliac
artery, the proximal end of the graft may be more conveniently sutured to the
side of the common iliac artery.

End-to-side anastomosis is then done to the external iliac artery just above the inguinal ligament, or to the common femoral via a one-finger tunnel under the inguinal ligament (Fig. 8-3).

In closing the oblique incision, it is most important that the fascia transversalis be clearly identified and carefully closed with running chromic catgut. Treat the internal oblique muscle similarly. Close the external oblique fascia with interrupted sutures. No drainage is needed.

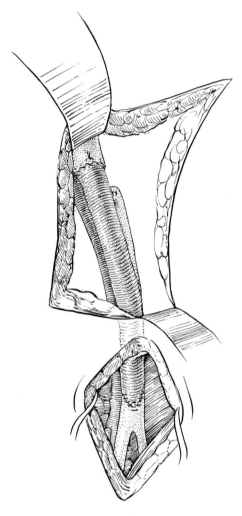

Figure 8-3.   Lower anastomosis, side-to-side to common femoral artery.

THROMBOSIS AFTER BRACHIAL ARTERY CATHETERIZATION

From the current widespread use of intraarterial catheters for diagnosis and therapy, the syndrome of postcatheterization thrombosis has emerged as an all-too-familiar phenomenon. Although it occurs in a minority of such procedures, its repair occupies a definite place on the operating room schedule of any hospital using modern radiologic or cardiologic diagnosis.

DIAGNOSIS

Do not wait for ischemia symptoms. After each procedure, determine the presence of distal pulsations by palpation or, if subcutaneous pulses cannot be felt, by oscillations or ultrasound or both. Assessed by any of these methods, pulsatile flow that is detectably less than it was preoperatively, with the diminution in pulsation persisting on a repeat examination, is diagnostic of thrombosis.

INDICATIONS

The presence of ischemia symptoms of a degree to threaten loss of tissue makes operation mandatory.

   In the extremity in which survival seems assured due to adequate collateral circulation, operative restoration of normal flow is nevertheless indicated in most cases. This is because in the early stages one cannot make a definitive assessment of the degree of chronic ischemia or the disability caused by it.

CONTRAINDICATIONS

Operation must be abandoned or postponed in these patients if a higher-priority consideration, such as treatment of cardiac failure or patient fatigue from a long procedure, so indicates.

PLANNING AND PREPARATION

No arteriogram is necessary.

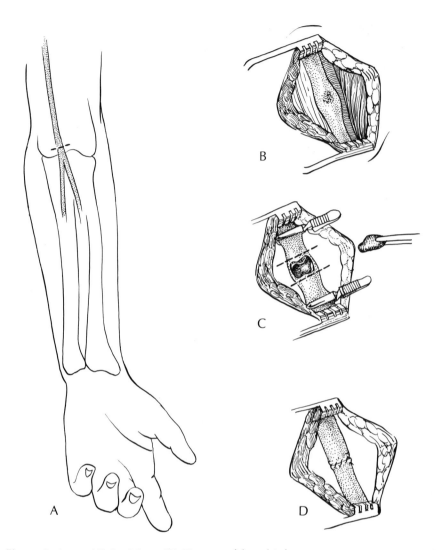

Figure 8-4.   (A) Incision. (B) Damaged brachial artery at puncture site. (C) Thrombectomy and resection of damaged segment. (D) End-to-end anastomosis.

OPERATION

Anesthesia: Use general or brachial block anesthesia.
Drape so that the hand can be examined by a nonsterile assistant.

Incision: Reopen and elongate the transverse incision used for the catheterization (Fig. 8-4A). If the catheterization was by percutaneous puncture, make the incision longitudinally over the artery at that site.

Procedure: After applying bulldog clamps, open the arteriotomy and remove the thrombus with manual extrusion and the Fogarty catheter distally (Fig. 8-4C). Instill heparin solution via an irrigating catheter before closing the artery.

Examine the artery at the site of injury to decide whether or not damage to its wall is sufficient to require resection. Frayed adventitia and detached or ragged intima indicate resection. The extent of this resection is rarely more than 5 mm. (Fig. 8-4C).

Perform end-to-end anastomosis with 5-0 Teflon (Fig. 8-4D).

In patients seen several days or weeks after thrombosis, arteriography is mandatory and catheter thrombectomy ineffective. The pattern of arterial obstruction is usually ideal for a brachiobrachial or a brachioradial bypass vein graft.

9   Immediate repair of arterial wounds

OBJECTIVE

To restore arterial circulation and to control hemorrhage.

INDICATIONS

Arterial repair is indicated when loss of the artery will cause immediate or long-term ischemia symptoms. The treatment of hemorrhage from smaller arteries is ligation.

Hemorrhage continuing in the form of external hemorrhage or an expanding, pulsating subcutaneous hematoma.

Ischemia of the part. The circulation is appraised by examination of the pulses, oscillations, and peripheral blood pressures. Absence of sensation, provided there is no nerve injury, is the best single indication of the nonviability of an ischemic limb. Others are listed on page 89.

If neither active hemorrhage nor ischemia is present and the wound requires debridement in the area of the lacerated artery, repair of the artery should be done as part of the debridement.

CONTRAINDICATIONS

None.

PLANNING AND PREPARATION

Examination for concomitant nerve injury is essential. This occurs in more than 50% of arterial injuries and is more frequent in the upper than in the lower extremity.

If doubt exists as to the level or extent of arterial injury and active hemorrhage is not an issue, perform arteriography.

OPERATION

Arrange for proximal control of the major trunk, if necessary through a separate incision (Fig. 9-1). Distal control is also desirable but is less important than proximal control.

Use a tourniquet if the wound is far enough distal on the limb.

Do not attempt to apply hemostatic forceps to a gushing arterial bleeder until the actual opening in the artery is visualized. Otherwise, nerve damage can easily result. With proximal control of the artery bleeding pressure is low, and gentle tamponade of the opening by the fingertip permits local dissection under adequate visualization.

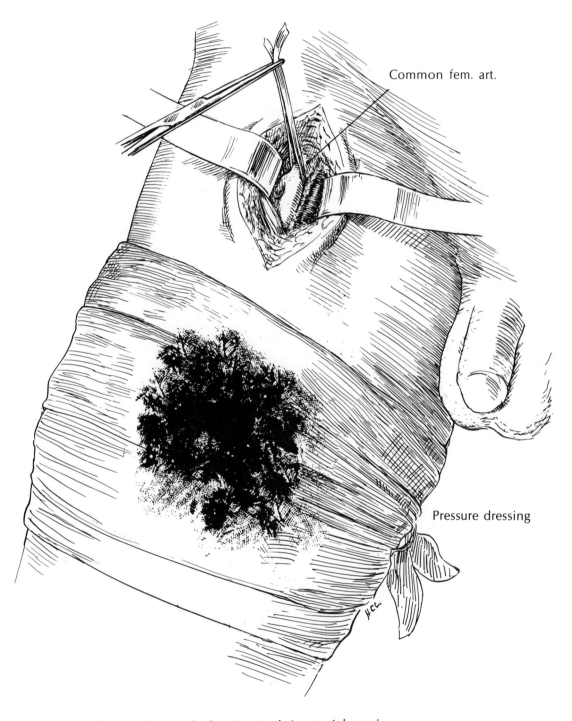

Common fem. art.

Pressure dressing

Figure 9-1.   Proximal control of major trunk in arterial repair.

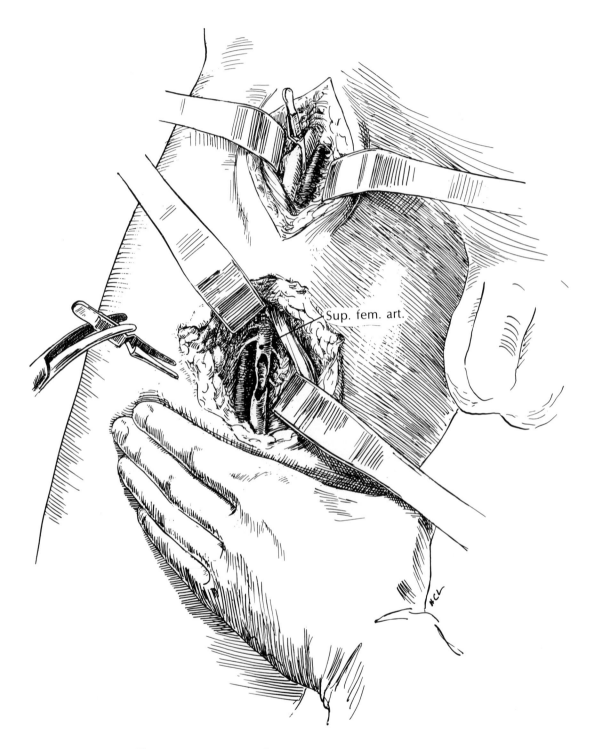

Figure 9-2.   Hemorrhage controlled, hematoma evacuated.

If these maneuvers are unsuccessful, full proximal and distal control of hemorrhage can often be accomplished by manual control, either externally (Fig. 9-2) or in the wound. The latter is effected by pulling the artery forward, using the fingers inserted behind it (see Fig. 10-2).

Apply arterial clamps at least 2 cm. from the ends to be sutured. Apply bulldog clamps to the branches.

Do not hesitate to sacrifice small branches in order to effect approximation. Do not sacrifice large ones, such as the deep femoral, circumflex femoral, deep brachial, or hypogastric artery.

Division and end-to-end suture with the trimmed ends cut somewhat obliquely are often better than lateral suture of a jagged hole in the artery (Fig. 9-3).

High-velocity missiles cause extensive arterial damage, and a graft is often needed in missile wounds. If so, use a segment of the saphenous vein (Fig. 9-4).

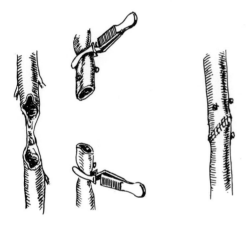

Figure 9-3.   Resection of severe laceration and direct end-to-end suture.

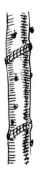

Figure 9-4.   Autogenous saphenous vein graft.

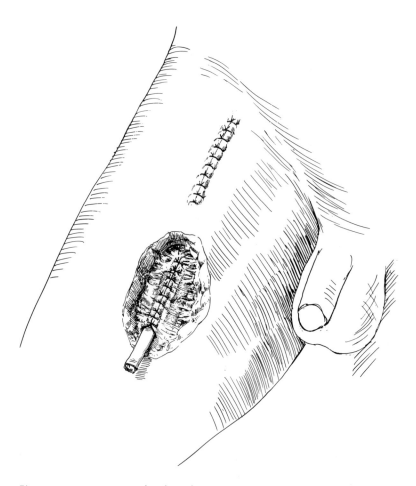

Figure 9-5.   Wounds closed.

Give 7500 units of heparin intravenously.

Repair concomitant injury to the major vein, if possible.

Close the muscle and fascia, at least, over an arterial repair. Debridement may make this difficult. It is then mandatory to sew a muscle flap to cover the repair. If repair has been delayed, leave the skin open and insert a deep drain for 24 hours (Fig. 9-5). A Hemovac is useful.

POSTOPERATIVE MANAGEMENT

An hourly check is made of pulses and oscillations until they are stable. If these disappear and the limb is in jeopardy, reexploration should be done immediately. If the limb is not in jeopardy, reoperation can be done at a later date as an elective procedure after arteriography.

10 Reconstruction for arteriovenous aneurysm (fistula)

OBJECTIVES

To avert or control heart failure, edema, ischemia, local hemorrhage, or bacterial endarteritis.

INDICATIONS

Operation is indicated for all traumatic arteriovenous aneurysms. They may increase in size, cause high-output heart failure and local complications (such as pain, nerve pressure, venous stasis, and external hemorrhage), and be the seat of bacterial infection.

Spontaneous aortocaval fistula results from the rupture of an aortic aneurysm into the inferior vena cava. In such a case, the need for operation is urgent.

Congenital arteriovenous aneurysms (cirsoid aneurysms) are operated on for cosmetic reasons or for symptoms. Symptoms are more likely to be local (bleeding, venous stasis problems) than to be those of cardiac failure, although high-output failure does occur with large defects. Operation for this type of aneurysm consists of multiple ligations or plastic excisions or both. Because of their diffuse nature, occasionally involving bone, removal often cannot be complete; but such aneurysms are not considered here.

CONTRAINDICATIONS

High-risk or intercurrent disease only.

PLANNING AND PREPARATION

The fistula is to be eliminated, preferably without interruption of arterial or venous circulation of the part.

In order of preference the methods that can be selected are:

1. Excision of the fistula and reconstruction of the artery and vein. This means local excision of the fistula plus lateral suture of the artery and vein, or excision of the fistula-bearing vessels followed by end-to-end suture or graft reconstruction of the artery.

2. Excision of the fistula and reconstruction of the artery but not the vein. The excluded vein may be used to aid lateral closure of the arterial opening.

3. Excision as above, without reconstruction of artery or vein.

4. "Quadruple ligation." This means ligation near the fistula of all afferent and efferent arteries and veins. Since it is difficult to isolate all feeding vessels without dissection to an equal or greater degree than is required for excision, quadruple ligation is not recommended.

In major arteries and veins, either procedure (1) or (2) is preferred. In many major arteries, such as the superficial femoral and external iliac, chronic ischemia symptoms often result unless arterial reconstruction is done.

In small arteries and veins, such as the posterior tibial artery, the forearm vessels, and the palmar arch, excision is the procedure of choice since no vascular impairment will result therefrom.

Never do proximal ligation of the artery alone! Since the distal hypotension due to the ligature is enhanced by loss of arterial pressure through the fistula, this procedure creates severe arterial stasis distal to the tie and gangrene may ensue.

Preoperative Study: Close the fistula by digital pressure and observe for bradycardia (Branham's sign) and for contraction of the pulse pressure.

Record the thrill and murmur.

Record the amount of dilatation of the afferent artery.

Perform arteriographic study routinely, not only to show the exact site of the fistula, but also to demonstrate the anatomic relationships and the afferent and efferent vessels.

Examine for local and systemic venous pressures, heart size (by x-ray), functional murmurs, and electrocardiographic abnormalities.

Timing: Wait six weeks after the onset of the fistula to allow development of collateral vessels, subsidence of local infection, and softening of scar tissue, unless the aneurysm is increasing in size or the fistula is of a magnitude to generate heart failure earlier than this.

OPERATION

The method in (1) above, which involves reconstruction of the artery and vein, is described.

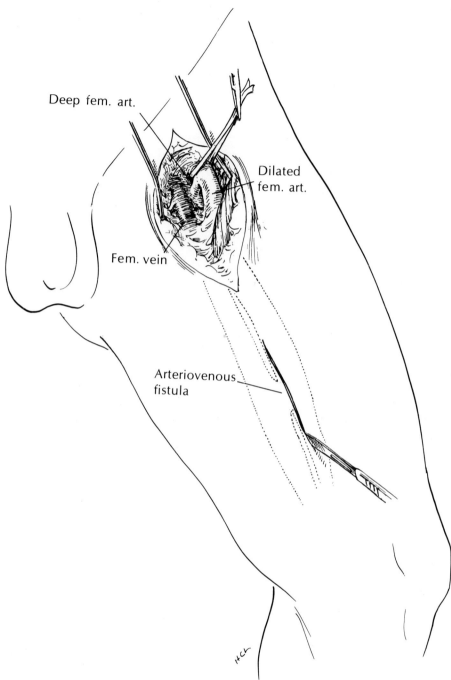

Figure 10-1.   Incision, proximal control.

Exposure: Provide wide exposure to allow early control of the principal afferent artery proximal to a point where any major abnormality exists (Fig. 10-1). If it is extremely dilated and thin-walled, potential control must be arranged proximal to this area, a maneuver that may occasionally take one back to the aorta.

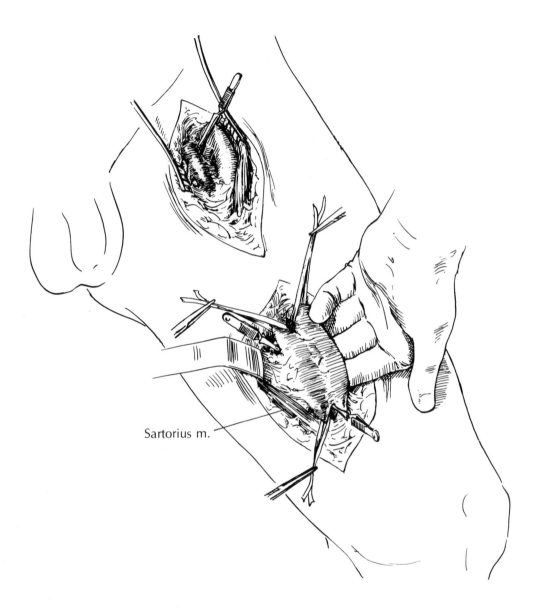

Sartorius m.

Figure 10-2.   Approach to lesion. Partial control with clamps; final control with fingers.

Dissection: Dissect all vessels supplying or draining the fistula and arrange for temporary closure thereof. If it is feared that all cannot be cleared without breaking into the vascular system, perform the dissection first deeply, so that the fingers can be introduced behind the fistula in order to lift it forward under tension (Fig. 10-2). Should bleeding occur, this will stop it and allow dissection to proceed.

Temporarily clamp all contributing vessels and divide the fistula (Fig. 10-3). At this point give 7500 units of heparin.

Reconstruction: Reconstruct the artery and vein. The degree of involvement by scar, and, to a lesser extent, the size of the fistula, will determine the method of reconstruction selected (Fig. 10-4).

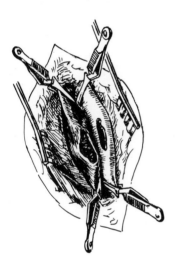

Figure 10-3.   Fistula divided and dissection completed.

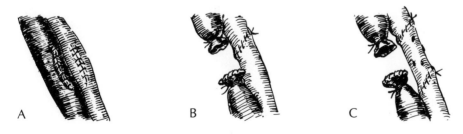

Figure 10-4.   Varieties of repair. (*A*) Lateral suture of vein and artery. (*B*) Resection of vein and anastomosis of artery. (*C*) Vein resection and vein graft replacement of artery.

POSTOPERATIVE MANAGEMENT

Heparin is not used.

NOTES ON REPAIR OF ARTERIOVENOUS
FISTULA RESULTING FROM RUPTURE OR AN
AORTIC ANEURYSM INTO THE
INFERIOR VENA CAVA

1.   Approach as in the case of a simple aortic aneurysm by obtaining control of the aorta above and the iliac arteries below.

2.   Avoid manipulation of the aneurysm, particularly after the clamps are applied, to prevent pulmonary embolism from the thrombus in the aneurysmal sac.

3.   If manipulation becomes necessary, temporarily occlude the fistula by pressure on the vena cava over it.

4.   Control of bleeding from the vena cava through the fistula into the opened aneurysm is not difficult. While the assistant's hands apply pressure on the vena cava above and below, close the lips of the fistula with an Allis forceps or a preliminary single suture.

5.   Definitively close the fistula after resection of most of the aneurysm sac by mattress sutures through the lips of the fistula: the adherent aorta and vena cava form a strong structure for this purpose.

II   Reconstruction for false (traumatic) arterial aneurysm

OBJECTIVE

To remove the risk of arterial hemorrhage and thrombosis and to repair the artery.

INDICATIONS

Traumatic aneurysms can enlarge or thrombose at any time, early or late, following their occurrence. They can also become infected and be the source of secondary hemorrhage. Operation is therefore indicated in all cases. If the artery is needed for normal limb circulation, it should be repaired; if not, it may be ligated.

If the blood clot is infected, the entire aneurysm sac, all clot, and a segment of artery surrounding the ostium must be excised. Autologous artery or vein graft is substituted, covered with muscle, and drained with a Hemovac for 24 hours.

The small aneurysms that occasionally result from femoral or brachial arteriograms can be operated on as soon as they are diagnosed.

CONTRAINDICATIONS

Severe intercurrent disease.

PLANNING AND PREPARATION

Provided the patient has access to competent surgical care, operation on an established false aneurysm that is not increasing in size and is not infected should be postponed until maximum softening of scar tissue has occurred. This requires one to three months after wounding.

Surgery should be undertaken early on an aneurysm that is painful, causing nerve pressure, increasing in size, or interfering with joint function.

Arteriography should be done routinely.

OPERATION

The steps are similar to those in repair of arteriovenous fistula (pp. 109–111). Do not persist in attempts to excise the aneurysm intact. It is wiser to break into it after its main supply has been controlled. If there is doubt about the presence of infection, make a gram stain of a smear of the clot and the arterial wall. This will dictate the use or nonuse of a graft if there is anything approaching an even choice.

Control is accomplished by one or more of three methods: (1) by surgical exposure and occlusion of the proximal and distal main arterial trunks and branches (Figs. 11-1 and 11-2); (2) by a tourniquet; or (3) by manual elevation of the area within the wound (Fig. 11-3). In aneurysms that occur following angiographic puncture, distal control is not necessary.

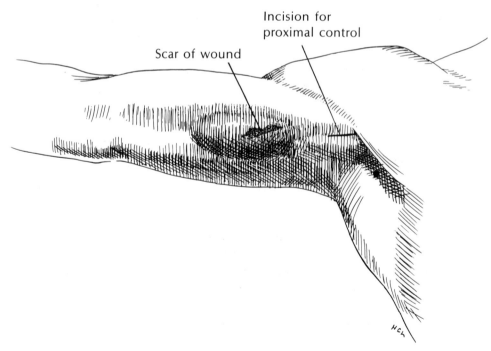

Incision for
proximal control

Scar of wound

Figure 11-1.   Skin incisions.

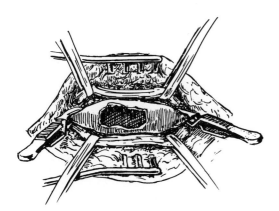

Figure 11-2.   Dissection completed.

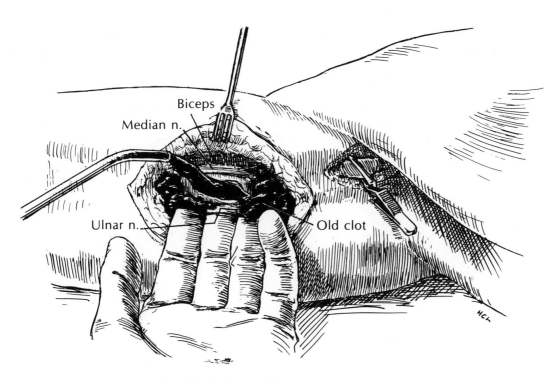

Figure 11-3.   Manual method of control.

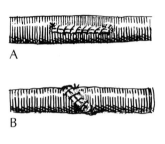

A

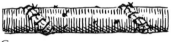

B

C

Figure 11-4.   Varieties of repair. (A) Simple suture. (B) End-to-end obliquely. (C) Vein graft.

If the hematoma cavity does not collapse, and if the smear is positive following turning out of the clot and arterial repair, a drain is left in, not touching the suture line. Three methods of arterial repair are shown in Figure 11-4.

POSTOPERATIVE MANAGEMENT

Heparin is not used.

An hourly check is made of pulses and oscillations until they are stable. If these disappear and the limb is in jeopardy, reexploration should be done immediately. If the limb is not in jeopardy, reexploration can be done at a later date as an elective procedure after arteriography.

12 Reconstruction for popliteal aneurysm

OBJECTIVE

To prevent thrombosis of the aneurysm, which usually results in gangrene of the foot.

To prevent embolism of fragments of clot or atheroma from the aneurysm sac down the tibial arteries. Repeated embolism gradually occludes these vessels, shutting down flow and finally causing thrombosis of the main sac.

The purposes of the bypass vein graft method are to permit early opening of the aneurysm sac, reduce dissection injury of adjacent structures, and maintain the integrity of knee joint function.

INDICATIONS

An aneurysm larger than 3 cm. in diameter.

An aneurysm smaller than 3 cm. in diameter, with loss of a pedal pulse.

Acute thrombosis, if seen within a few hours, with the fate of the limb in doubt.

Old thrombosis with a surviving but ischemic leg, if an arteriogram shows open vessels below.

CONTRAINDICATIONS

A thrombosed aneurysm in the absence of ischemia symptoms (rare).

A thrombosed aneurysm with gangrene already established.

PLANNING AND PREPARATION

Appraise the circulation.

Examine the opposite popliteal space (in 3 out of 4 cases popliteal aneurysms occur bilaterally), the femoral arteries, and the abdominal aorta for other aneurysms.

Perform an arteriogram to appraise the caliber and quality of the femoral artery above the aneurysm. Many have secondary sacculations or stenoses at the adductor canal. The origin of a bypass graft should be above any such pathologic condition.

Broad-spectrum antibiotics, administered intravenously, should be started 4 hours before operation and discontinued four days later.

OPERATION

Position: Supine, with leg somewhat everted and knee semiflexed over a folded gown.

Incisions: Medial infracondylar, 10 cm. long (Fig. 12-1), and medial supracondylar, 7 cm. long.

Make two incisions in the upper thigh, the first over the saphenous bulb and the second several centimeters below, in order to secure a suitable length of greater saphenous vein.

Make the medial supracondylar incision first just posterior to the femur, which is a constant guide, and anterior to the sartorius and the adductor tendon; deepen it to the upper popliteal artery and clear it for 6 cm. (Fig. 12-2A). Encircle it with a tape. Any pathologic condition seen in the arteriogram above the joint line should be identified as to level in the artery, so that the vein-graft takeoff can be suitably situated.

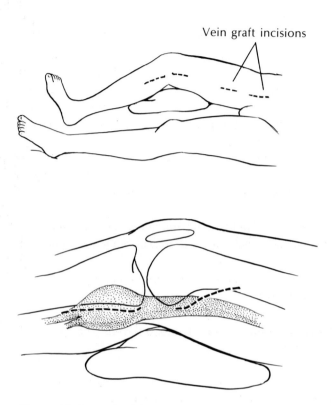

Vein graft incisions

Figure 12-1.   Incisions.

Dissection: With proximal control established, carry the infracondylar incision through the deep fascia just posterior to the posterior wall of the tibia and gradually clear the medial wall of the aneurysm. The popliteal vein will be securely bound to the medial aspect of the aneurysm sac on its ventral aspect. No attempt is made to free this junction. Just below the aneurysm the vein will be relatively free of the artery. At this point, dissect the popliteal artery to its bifurcation and encircle it with a tape.

Dissect all aspects of the aneurysm sac, but only to the extent that such dissection is easy, exposure is excellent, and any arterial or venous branches can be clearly visualized. The sciatic nerve, lying posterolaterally, is left alone.

Divide small branches of the popliteal vein ramifying over the aneurysm sac. Divide easily accessible geniculate or sural arterial branches coming off of the aneurysm sac.

Depending on the size and degree of adherence of the aneurysm, only the medial third of the sac may be dissected, or the entire circumference may be freed.

Obtain a suitable length of upper greater saphenous vein (see Chap. 5). Give 7500 units of heparin.

Resection of the Sac: Clamp the upper popliteal artery at the level of the adductor canal and the popliteal artery just above its bifurcation (Fig. 12-2B). Open the sac over its entire length (Fig. 12-2C). Remove mural clot and pack off backbleeding arterial branches from inside the sac. Then oversew these ostia as gauze or fingertip pressure is withdrawn. With the sac empty and collapsed, further blunt and sharp dissection may easily free more of it without injuring either the popliteal vein or muscular branches of the sciatic nerve. Ligate the popliteal artery just above the aneurysm (Fig. 12-2D).

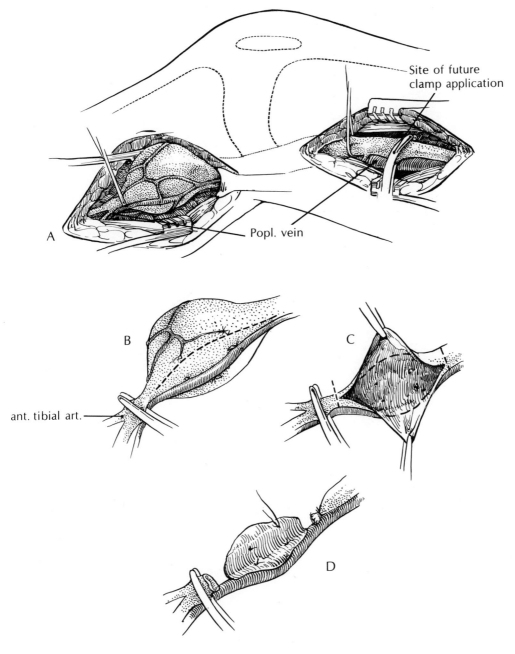

Figure 12-2.   (A) Proximal control. Dissecting the aneurysm. (B) Clamping the distal popliteal artery. (C) Opening the sac. (D) Trimming away excess sac and securing backbleeding vessels.

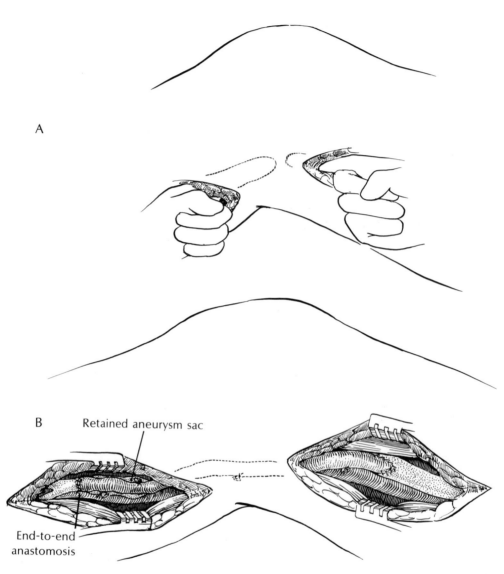

Figure 12-3.   (*A*) Opening the popliteal tunnel. (*B*) Bypass graft completed.

Now remove all freed portions of the sac. Transect the popliteal artery 1 cm. above the lower clamp. Use the index fingers of both hands against the ventromedial aspect of the artery to dissect open the popliteal tunnel (Fig. 12-3A).

Suture the proximal end of the saphenous vein end to end to the distal cut popliteal artery. Draw the graft up through the tunnel, distend it again to prevent twisting, and suture it end to side to the upper popliteal or lower superficial femoral artery above any significant disease (Fig. 12-3B). Irrigate the entire area and carefully search for any residual small bleeding points along the cut edge of the aneurysm sac.

It is well to drain the aneurysm cavity by a Hemovac suction line passing down from the supracondylar incision. Remove this tubing in 24 hours.

In the resection of a popliteal aneurysm, it is tempting to divide the adductor tendon, both hamstring tendons, and the origins of the gastrocnemius and soleus muscles about 5 mm. from their attachments to provide almost total exposure of the popliteal space. This is rarely necessary or desirable. Full rehabilitation in the sense of free ambulation without stiffness or discomfort is achieved very slowly after these more extensive procedures.

13 Thromboendarterectomy or bypass of the extracranial arterial circulation

OBJECTIVES

To restore mainstream arterial flow to the brain.

To prevent embolism to the brain from ulcerated atheroma.

To restore subclavian or vertebral pressure and flow. Rarely, in innominate artery stenosis, to restore pressure and flow to the right subclavian and carotid arteries.

INDICATIONS

Recurrent transient ischemia attacks with prompt recovery and no neurologic deficit, together with a demonstrated significant carotid bifurcation lesion, either stenosis or ulceration. Patients with minimal neurologic deficits may be considered for operation after a six weeks' wait, a period that greatly reduces the likelihood of postoperative stroke.

Hemispheric or monocular transient ischemia attacks, often reinforced by a carotid bifurcation bruit, indicate arteriography. If internal carotid stenosis of 50% or more or an ulcerated atheromatous plaque (often shown in oblique views) is present in the symptomatic circuit, surgical repair is indicated.

When bilateral carotid stenoses are accompanied by monocular or hemispheric symptoms, direct the surgical repair to the artery corresponding to the symptoms, even if it is less stenotic than its fellow. If the patient remains symptom free postoperatively, the opposite carotid will not often require operation unless the stenosis is significantly advanced (to a caliber of 1 to 2 mm.).

In patients with bilateral significant carotid stenoses presenting with verte-brobasilar symptoms, space the operative repairs of the carotids by four- to six-week intervals, whether or not vertebral artery stenosis is present. In patients who have had closure of one internal carotid and have 50% or more stenosis of the other together with transient ischemic attacks, whether lateralized or not, the stenotic lesion should be repaired.

In patients presenting with proximal stenosis of the innominate or carotid trunks, in those with proximal subclavian stenosis, and in those with vertebral artery stenoses, cerebral infarction does not develop in the absence of additional carotid bifurcation stenoses. If internal carotid stenosis coexists with the preceding lesions, repair of the internal carotid lesion will prevent stroke.

Where convincing symptoms correspond to a well-demonstrated subclavian steal syndrome, a carotid-to-subclavian bypass in the neck is indicated, provided the internal carotid arteries are free of significant stenoses.

Rarely, arm claudication without central nervous system symptoms warrants carotid-to-subclavian bypass.

CONTRAINDICATIONS

Patients with complete obstruction of the internal carotid artery, whether acute or chronic (exception: acute closure during angiography).

Unilateral stenosis of a vertebral artery, whether or not accompanied by carotid stenosis.

Incidentally discovered asymptomatic stenosis in any of the extracranial arteries, except in the instance of a 1- to 2-mm. carotid stenosis in a patient needing another elective major operation.

PLANNING AND PREPARATION

A neurologist should be requested to see all patients in consultation.

In most instances, arteriography should be performed by the retrograde femoral route to include aortic arch injections, selective carotid and vertebral views, and oblique views. Usually, make studies of the intracranial vessels to rule out tumor or other critical abnormalities and to show crossover competence of the circle of Willis.

Consider special studies, such as ophthalmodynamometry, electroencephalography, or brain scans where indicated.

STENOSIS OF THE CAROTID BIFURCATION OR INTERNAL CAROTID ARTERY

OPERATION

Position: Supine, with the headrest dropped slightly and a small pillow between the shoulders to hyperextend the neck. The face is rotated sharply away from the lesion.

Anesthesia: General endotracheal. Place a Mayo stand just above the patient's face to support the drapes. The anesthesiologist sits at the patient's side. Thus the surgical team can stand at any point around the patient's head or at either side of the neck for excellent access.

Place an intravenous line for the ready administration of any needed drug. Use a Javid shunt in every case, so that the adequacy of cerebral blood flow during operation is never in doubt.

Incision: Follow the anterior border of the sternocleidomastoid muscle (Fig. 13-1), starting 1 cm. below the angle of the mandible.

Dissection: As the incision is deepened through the platysma muscle and the sternocleidomastoid muscle is retracted laterally, the pulsation of the common carotid artery is readily detected. Open the carotid sheath, draw the vagus nerve posteriorly with the jugular vein, and dissect the common carotid artery upward to its bifurcation.

Identify the external carotid artery by its first two anterior branches, the superior thyroid and the lingual. Divide and ligate the superior thyroid artery to permit subsequent easy elevation and circumferential dissection of the external carotid takeoff.

Dissect the internal carotid artery as far as possible superiorly. This artery is branchless in the neck and lies posterior and lateral to the external carotid.

Isolate and preserve the hypoglossal nerve crossing both carotids just at the origin of the occipital branch of the external carotid. At the uppermost margin of the incision next to the mandible, care should be taken to preserve the mandibular branch of the facial nerve.

The fine nervous filament representing the descending branch of the hypoglossal nerve will be found lying either anterior to the carotid sheath or right

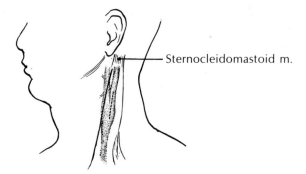

Sternocleidomastoid m.

Figure 13-1.   Incision.

on top of the artery itself. At the lower end of the dissection, note the narrow omohyoid muscle belly or tendon.

When either a highly occlusive plaque or an ulcerated atheroma is detected at the bifurcation, it is important not to palpate the lesion vigorously or to kink it by sharp elevation with a tape.

The great protection afforded by an internal shunt requires wide dissection of both the internal and the common carotid arteries so that at least 2.5 cm. of vessel is completely cleared above and below the upper and lower margins of the lesion.

Give 7500 units of heparin intravenously.

Placing the Shunt: Clamp the external carotid artery 1 cm. away from the bifurcation. Place gentle traction on the tape around the internal carotid artery, which has been freed well above the hypoglossal nerve, and apply a vascular clamp as high as possible. The common carotid artery is then clamped well down below the plaque.

Using a small blade, open the anterior wall of the common carotid artery just below the plaque. Cut through the artery and plaque with a Potts scissors for a distance of 1 cm. above and below the margins of the stenotic lesion so that normal intima is well seen. Place stay sutures to hold the arteriotomy open (Fig. 13-2B).

Insert the small end of the shunt into the internal carotid artery, making sure that it is not too large and that the intima is not stripped (Fig. 13-2B). Remove the upper vascular clamp with the shunt tubing compressed while the shunt is advanced another 1 cm. into the internal carotid and the Javid internal carotid clamp is placed below the flange on the shunt, as in Figure 13-2C. Allow the shunt to fill completely with blood so that all the air is displaced. Then clamp it. Direct the larger end of the shunt into the common carotid as the vascular clamp is slightly and momentarily released to displace with blood any air trapped between the shunt and the clamp.

Advance the shunt 2.5 cm. into the common carotid, apply the larger Javid clamp above the shoulder of the shunt, and remove the vascular clamp (Fig. 13-2C).

These steps involving shunt placement should be well rehearsed so that less than 2 minutes is needed to establish flow through it.

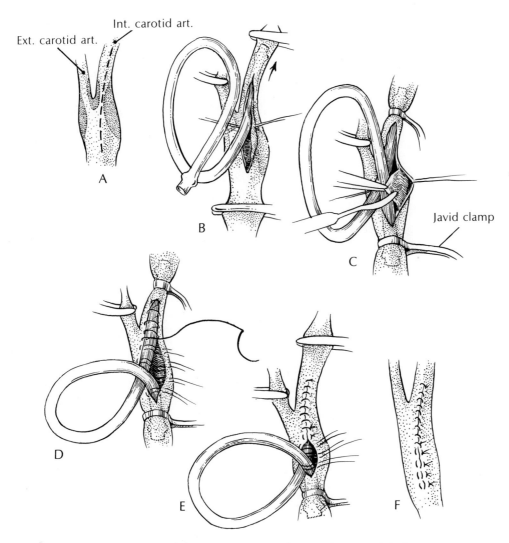

Figure 13-2.   (A) Carotid arteriotomy. (B) Placing the internal shunt. (C) Beginning the endarterectomy. (D) Beginning closure of the arteriotomy. (E) Removing the shunt. (F) Endarterectomy completed.

The Endarterectomy: Perform endarterectomy with the shunt in place, usually beginning at a point near the center of the anteriotomy where the loose plane in the media is most evident (Fig. 13-2C). After this dissection has been carried completely around the artery, cut across the plaque and dissect the two halves free separately.

The upper half contains the atheromatous projections into the external and internal carotid arteries. With the internal carotid open beyond the atheroma, it is usually easier to dissect this segment of the plaque next, using a narrow spud or dissector. This segment of the core terminates either as a very thin cylindrical cuff or as a narrowing tongue of atheroma tapering into normal intima. It is imperative that no shelf or dissection plane be left. In the rare event that a shelf is unavoidable, tack the thickened edge down by interrupted sutures.

With the upper core free except for the external carotid component, it is easy to obtain circumferential dissection of this extension with the tip of the dissector visible through the arterial wall.

The lower half of the divided plaque is freed only a short distance into the common carotid artery, because the intimal thickening tends to extend proximally for long distances. The core is cut off with sharp scissors. It is unnecessary to tack down the remaining shelf.

After removal of the atheroma, gently scrub the lining of the carotid artery with a small pledget held in a right-angled clamp to clear out loose shreds or odd bits of atheroma. The area is freely irrigated with saline.

By displacing both limbs of the shunt inferiorly, close the upper 2 cm. of the arteriotomy with a running 5-0 suture. Four mattress sutures are then laid in place on either side of the shunt tubing for easy closure of the lower 1.5 cm. of the arteriotomy later on. (For convenience, these steps are combined in Figure 13-2D).

Now clamp the free loop of the shunt and withdraw the internal carotid limb after removing the Javid clamp. Allow the internal carotid to backbleed momentarily before a vascular clamp is applied. Remove the common carotid clamp and shunt after applying a vascular clamp (Fig. 13-2E). The four mattress sutures are then tied. Remove the clamp on the external carotid artery to expel residual air through the suture line while the artery fills with blood. Next, remove the common carotid clamp so that any residual air bubbles or bits of vascular debris will pass harmlessly into the external carotid artery. The clamp on the internal carotid is removed last (Fig. 13-2F). If diffuse oozing is present, give protamine sulfate.

Close the carotid sheath over the repaired artery with interrupted sutures. Close the platysma and skin in two layers over a Hemovac drain, which is removed in 24 hours.

CAROTID-TO-SUBCLAVIAN BYPASS
FOR INNOMINATE OR SUBCLAVIAN
ARTERY STENOSIS

OBJECTIVES

To restore flow to the innominate or subclavian artery.

INDICATIONS

Subclavian steal syndrome. For the considerations involved in deciding which operation to use for subclavian steal syndrome, see page 135.

OPERATION

Position: Supine, face turned to the opposite side and ipsilateral arm at the side in order not to elevate the clavicle.

Incision: Transverse, just above the clavicle, from the anterior midline of the neck to the midpoint of the clavicle (Fig. 13-3).

Dissection: Deepen the incision through the platysma muscle and the deep cervical fascia and divide much of the clavicular origin of the sternocleido-mastoid muscle. Displace the subclavian vein downward and, as the carotid sheath is opened, retract the jugular vein and the vagus nerve medially.

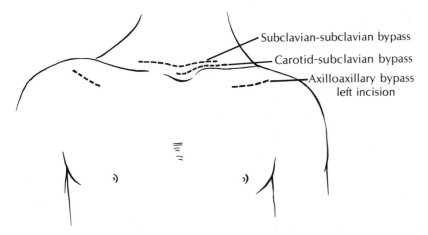

Subclavian-subclavian bypass
Carotid-subclavian bypass
Axilloaxillary bypass
left incision

Figure 13-3.   Incisions for bypasses.

Between the subclavian vein and artery the anterior scalene muscle comes into view. This is the key to the dissection, as this muscle covers the apex of the subclavian loop. After identifying and protecting the phrenic nerve on its anterolateral surface, divide its tendinous insertion into the scalene tubercle of the first rib with shallow sweeps of a knife while a partly opened right-angled clamp protects the artery on the deep side. As the muscle retracts upward, the artery comes into view. It is easily cleared. Encircle it with a tape and dissect it free for 3 to 4 cm.

At times it is convenient to divide and ligate either the internal mammary artery or the thyrocervical trunk, or both, to gain helpful mobility of the subclavian loop.

Free the carotid artery from its sheath over a distance of 3 to 4 cm. by retracting the sternocleidomastoid muscle toward the midline and drawing the artery out from under the muscle.

Preclot a 10-mm. Dacron graft.

Give 7500 units of heparin.

Placing the Graft: Draw the lateral aspect of the common carotid artery into a curved clamp and make an arteriotomy and end-to-side anastomosis (Fig. 13-4A). Then clamp the graft next to the anastomosis and remove the vascular clamp from the carotid.

Cut the distal end of the graft at a 45-degree angle so that it will fit the top of the subclavian artery loop properly, and carry out end-to-side anastomosis to the superior aspect of this vessel. Remove both clamps, first removing that on the graft.

For those rare instances of innominate artery stenosis, see Figure 13-4B.

Close the incision in layers over a Hemovac drain left beneath the deep fascia for 24 hours.

SUBCLAVIAN-TO-CAROTID BYPASS FOR CAROTID ARTERY STENOSIS

OBJECTIVE

To restore common carotid pressure and flow.

INDICATIONS

Transient ischemia attacks referable to an advanced stenosis of the corresponding common carotid artery.

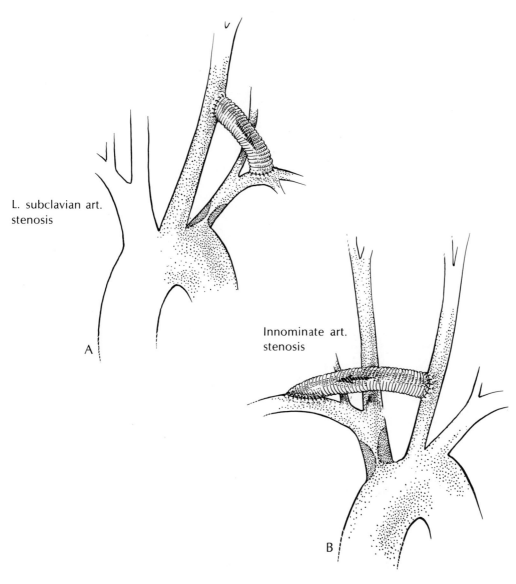

L. subclavian art.
stenosis

Innominate art.
stenosis

A

B

Figure 13-4.   (A) Carotid-to-subclavian bypass for subclavian stenosis. (B)
Carotid-to-subclavian bypass for innominate artery stenosis.

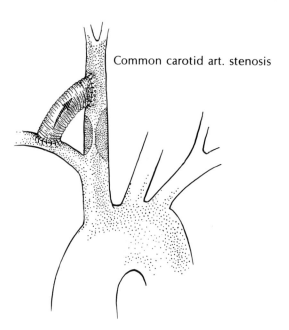

Figure 13-5.   Subclavian-to-carotid bypass.

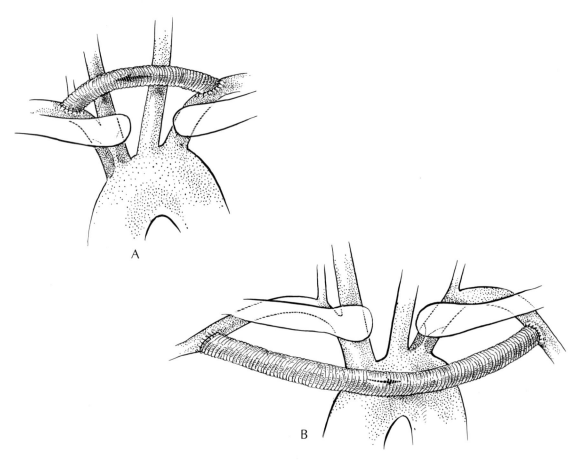

Figure 13-6.   (A) Subclavian-to-subclavian bypass. (B) Axilloaxillary bypass.

OPERATION

This operation is, of course, identical to that for the subclavian steal syndrome except that blood flow through the graft is in the opposite direction (Fig. 13-5).

SUBCLAVIAN-TO-SUBCLAVIAN BYPASS AND AXILLOAXILLARY BYPASS FOR INNOMINATE OR SUBCLAVIAN ARTERY STENOSIS

OBJECTIVES

To restore innominate or subclavian pressure and flow.

INDICATIONS

Subclavian steal syndrome; rarely, for carotid artery insufficiency in the case of an innominate artery stenosis.

OPERATION

Despite the remote chance of creating a steal situation by grafting from a normal carotid artery, some surgeons prefer to secure bypass inflow from an arm artery rather than from a carotid artery. For both the short and long term, the operation of subclavian-to-subclavian bypass depicted in Figure 13-6A appears to be safer than bypass from a common carotid to the opposite subclavian, as shown in Figure 13-4B.

For the axilloaxillary bypass, the incisions and axillary artery dissections are exactly as described for axillofemoral bypass (Chap. 4). A 10-mm. Dacron graft is placed in a subcutaneous tunnel that crosses the lower manubrium at the level of the second rib (Fig. 13-6B).

14 Renal artery reconstruction for stenosis

OBJECTIVES

To cure or improve hypertension.
   To improve total renal clearance when it is borderline or reduced.
   To prevent autonephrectomy by thrombosis of an advanced stenosis.
   To prevent hypertensive crisis.

INDICATIONS

Diastolic hypertension (defined as diastolic pressure over 100 mm. Hg.) when shown to be caused by renal artery stenosis.

CONTRAINDICATIONS

Stenosis not producing a pressure gradient.
   Uncontrolled hypertension at the time of planned operation.
   Late renal failure.

PLANNING AND PREPARATION

The diagnosis is usually suggested by the sudden first appearance of hypertension or the rapid acceleration of preexisting hypertension.

   The first screening test, an intravenous pyelogram, shows the involved kidney to be at least 1.5 cm. shorter than the normal one, with delayed function and hyperconcentration of contrast medium on the involved side.

   In most cases, the aortogram shows a convincing single advanced stenosis with a 1- to 2-mm. lumen and poststenotic dilatation. Such a lesion at or close to the renal artery ostium represents a circumferential atheroma. Farther out on the artery it can be due to subintimal fibrosis or an old stretch injury. The "string-of-beads" appearance of fibromuscular hyperplasia is unmistakable. The condition predominates in females by a ratio of 8 to 1 and usually occurs on the right, but it is bilateral in a third of the cases. In fibromuscular disease the total effect of the multiple lesions on distal renal artery pressure is often difficult to estimate from the arteriogram; under these circumstances, test for renal vein renin levels.

If there is doubt as to the importance of any stenosis, obtain renal vein renin levels; a 2 to 1 ratio favoring the involved side is diagnostic. However, if the stenotic lumen measures 2 mm. or less, this finding takes precedence over the renin level report.

Perform bilateral 10-minute ureteral urine sampling (Howard or Stamey test) for volume, osmolarity, and sodium content when stenosis is bilateral, when total renal clearance is impaired, or when the pathologic picture is mixed, e.g., old pyelonephritis plus stenosis.

The patient should understand that successful reconstruction of a renal artery cannot be guaranteed and that there is a small chance nephrectomy will be necessary. Nephrectomy is the procedure of choice when the renal mass is small (less than 8 to 9 cm.) or when function of the involved kidney is minimal because of nonvascular disease.

Occasional patients are seen in whom aortography shows that an arteriosclerotic stenosis has thrombosed and is occluding the main renal artery next to the aorta, but the distal artery and its subdivisions fill with dye via capsular, adrenal, and lumbar collaterals. The nephrogram is faint and urine excretion minimal. In such cases, endarterectomy with thrombectomy or an aortorenal bypass graft dramatically improves hypertension and renal function, often over weeks, as arteriolosclerosis gradually reverses.

Control hypertension prior to and during operation by 0.1% trimethaphan camsylate (Arfonad) drip if necessary to keep the diastolic pressure under 100 mm. Hg. At very high pressures, arterial anastomoses leak profusely between sutures and through suture holes.

Give 1000 ml. of 5% dextrose in water intravenously prior to induction of anesthesia to ensure high urine volumes during operation. Place a nasogastric tube.

Because of late stenosis or aneurysm formation in aortorenal saphenous vein grafts, the best graft appears to be the hypogastric artery, with an 8-mm. Dacron prosthesis as the second choice. In atherosclerotic patients, renal angiographic study should include the hypogastric arteries, which may be too diseased to use. Always include access to one saphenous vein in the prepared field.

OPERATION

Position: Supine.

Incision and Exposure: The choice of incision is between a long subcostal and a high midline or paramedian (Fig. 14-1). The long subcostal, which crosses the midline for 2.5 cm., gives excellent exposure of the renal artery, aorta, and corresponding kidney. It is ideal for a unilateral operation, includ-

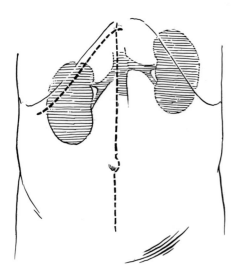

Figure 14-1.   Incisions.

ing renal biopsy, when endarterectomy or aortorenal bypass using a saphenous vein or an 8-mm. Dacron graft is planned. For bilateral procedures, or
when the hypogastric artery is to be used for a graft, the long midline or
paramedian incision is mandatory.

When using the subcostal incision on the right, open the peritoneum,
retract the transverse colon downward, and free up and reflect the duodenal
loop to the patient's left, exposing the right renal vein, vena cava, and nearby
structures. When using this incision on the left, open the peritoneum and the
peritoneal reflection of the descending colon widely. With Deaver retractors
reflecting the left colon to the right, the left renal vein, juxtaposed aorta, and
vena cava are exposed.

When a midline or long paramedian incision is used for bilateral renal
artery procedures, the exposure is the same as for aortic aneurysm (Chap. 1).

General Rules of Procedure: These are as follows.

1.   Leave the kidney in its bed in order to maintain capsular blood flow.
When function is poor in mixed disease, take a renal biopsy. This may point
to nephrectomy.

2.   Dissect the renal vein first, including complete clearing of its junction
with the vena cava and circumferential dissection of the vena cava for 2 to 3
cm. above and below the renal vein.

3.   Divide and ligate the gonadal vein on the left and the inferior adrenal
vein on either side. Do not use clips on any of these veins; they would be
scraped off by retractors.

4. With the renal vein retracted cephalad, dissect the artery, starting near its primary division and including 1 to 2 cm. of the major branches, and clear it to the aorta. On the right it may be necessary to divide one or two pairs of lumbar veins to free up the vena cava. If endarterectomy is planned, the nearby aorta must be completely cleared and the closest lumbar artery divided so that a clamp taking a side bite of aorta to exclude the renal artery takeoff will include one-half of the aortic circumference (Fig. 14-2A). The endarterectomy must include the rim of atheroma that lies within the aorta (Fig. 14-2B).

5. Give 7500 units of heparin prior to crossclamping the renal artery.

6. Although the renal artery usually can be clamped for 40 minutes with impunity, try to keep the time under 20 minutes. The more advanced the stenosis, the greater the leeway. If events portend the prolongation of warm ischemia time, perfuse the renal artery via sterile intravenous tubing with a unit of blood that has been packed in slush ice.

7. Give furosemide (Lasix) or mannitol prior to crossclamping if urine output is less than 50 ml. per hour.

8. In aortorenal bypass, divide one pair of lumbar arteries just above the inferior mesenteric artery takeoff so that the aorta can be lifted free. Properly applied at this level of aorta, an excluding clamp should be completely occlusive. Otherwise, the edges of the aortotomy protruding from the clamp will be too narrow for easy suturing. Do the end-to-side renal artery anastomosis first. Then place a small bulldog clamp on the graft next to the anastomosis and remove the renal artery clamp so that flow to the kidney can be promptly restored. Excise a 10 × 3 mm. ovoid segment from the right anterolateral aortic wall or the left midlateral aortic wall, as the case may be.

9. In right-sided aortorenal bypass, place the graft so that it lies anterior to the vena cava.

Thromboendarterectomy: Endarterectomy is the simplest procedure for atheromatous lesions. If the clamp or clamps that exclude the renal artery ostium from aortic blood flow allow ample access to the intra-aortic rim of plaque (Fig. 14-2B), and if full dissection of the renal vein, renal artery, and nearby aorta give excellent exposure, removal of the obstructing atheroma can be carried out much as it is in the carotid artery. The outer media and adventitia of the carotid artery, however, are invariably of good quality, whereas the renal artery in the hypertensive patient may be paper-thin outside the plaque itself and very friable. Occasionally the adventitia disrupts posteriorly, and the procedure has to be abandoned in favor of reimplantation of the renal artery into the aorta or an interposition graft. Such unplanned maneuvers add markedly to crossclamping time. In general, aortorenal bypass is safer. However, when the aorta is seen on the arteriogram to be heavily calcified and irregularly ulcerated and the yellow color of the stenotic

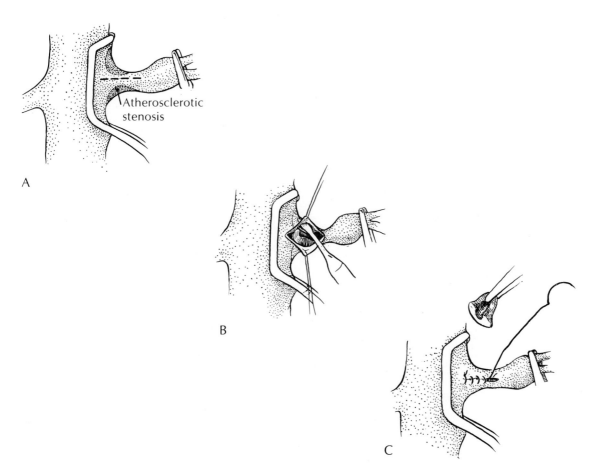

Figure 14-2.   (A) Approach to an atherosclerotic stenosis. (B) Thrombo-endarterectomy of the renal artery begun. (C) Thromboendarterectomy completed.

atheroma is not visible through the adventitia of the renal artery, choose endarterectomy over aortorenal bypass.

Aortorenal Bypass: In aortorenal bypass the preferable graft appears to be the hypogastric artery, provided this vessel is normal or nearly so. In obtaining the maximum length of this artery, free up 1 cm. of superior gluteal artery so that this first branch can be separately ligated and divided. Dissect an additional 1 cm. or so of hypogastric artery distally to gain additional length. The artery is then swung out on mild tension, and an excluding clamp is placed on the iliac artery in such a way that the hypogastric artery can be cut with sharp scissors exactly at its base. Close the resulting sidewall defect in the iliac artery with a running suture.

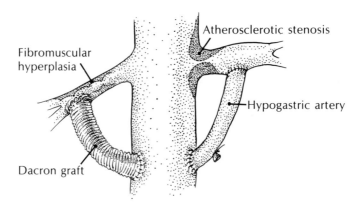

Figure 14-3.   Dacron bypass graft to the right renal artery for fibromuscular hyperplasia and bypass graft to the left renal artery, using hypogastric artery.

When grafting to a poststenotic dilatation, as in Figure 14-3 (left side), all sutures must be placed and drawn through the artery wall carefully and handled with minimum traction. This thinned-out wall is at times soft and holds sutures poorly. Occasionally it is wise to abandon the end-to-side anastomosis, especially with a Y-graft in which the aortic end of the graft is already in place. Most of the poststenotic dilatation can be excised obliquely, making possible a better-quality oblique end-to-end anastomosis to the distal artery. (For completeness, a Dacron bypass in a patient with fibromuscular dysplasia is shown on the right side in Figure 14-3.)

Figure 14-4 shows the aortic takeoff of a Y-graft just above the bifurcation. If this area is the site of marked atheromatous change, place the aortic anastomosis just 3 to 4 cm. below the renal arteries. It is better, however, to anastomose an 8-mm. Dacron graft end to side from one renal artery to the other in order to cross the aorta at this level, and then to join the anterior wall of the aorta to the posterior aspect of the graft with a 2-cm. segment of 10-mm. Dacron (Fig. 14-5). This creates an arterial distribution much like the celiac axis. It tends to lie without kinking better than does a broadened-out Y-graft.

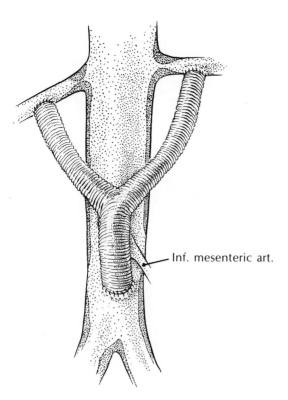

Figure 14-4.   Bilateral aortorenal Y-graft.

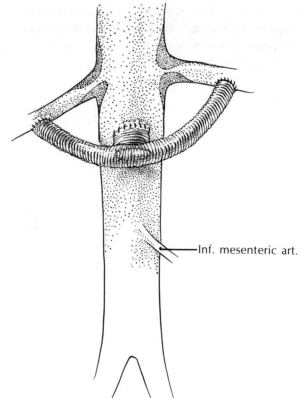

Figure 14-5.   Bilateral composite aortorenal Y-graft.

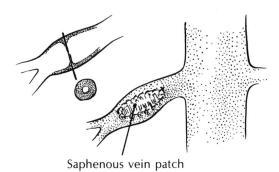

Saphenous vein patch

Figure 14-6.   Vein patch repair.

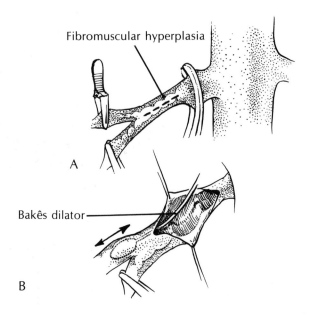

Fibromuscular hyperplasia

A

Bakês dilator

B

Figure 14-7.   (*A*) Arteriotomy for fibromuscular hyperplasia. (*B*) Dilation of renal artery branches.

Occasional patients have a very short, localized stenosis in the middle third of the renal artery caused by subintimal or medial fibrosis of unknown cause. A saphenous vein patch provides an ideal technical solution (Fig. 14-6).

Make a 2-cm. axial arteriotomy centered on the lesion. If the stenosis is less than 2 mm. in diameter, its circumference, when opened out, will obviously measure less than 6 mm. Trim an ovoid saphenous vein patch so that it measures 2.4 × 1.4 cm. when gently stretched. Such a patch will adequately open up the stenotic segment without creating an aneurysm.

Do not use segments of ovarian vein or vena cava for such a patch. They will eventually rupture under arterial pressure.

In fibromuscular hyperplasia affecting the first renal artery subdivisions, dilate these branches gently and gradually through an 8-mm. longitudinal arteriotomy in the distal renal artery (Fig. 14-7). Use small dilators or mosquito hemostats. If the main renal artery is also involved with the same process, suture a bypass graft to this arteriotomy.

POSTOPERATIVE MANAGEMENT

At 48 hours, obtain an intravenous pyelogram to be sure that the arterial reconstruction is functioning. If the radiographic dye is visible in faint concentration (especially after prolonged renal artery crossclamping), obtain a renal scan. This will differentiate between failure of the reconstruction and transient ischemic injury with probable full recovery.

15 *Aortomesenteric or aortoceliac bypass*

To cure "intestinal angina."
   To prevent mesenteric thrombosis with intestinal necrosis.

INDICATIONS

The relationship between angiographically demonstrable stenoses of the superior mesenteric and celiac arteries and various abdominal pain syndromes is not clear. Patients can be entirely symptom free despite gradual complete closure of the takeoff of both the celiac axis and the superior mesenteric artery. The usefulness of treating such stenoses to avoid future acute intestinal necrosis, while not proved, is logical. Such controlling factors as speed of occlusion, extent of collateral buildup, and the maintained level of central aortic pressure are unpredictable.

Rare patients will be found in whom large meals regularly induce periumbilical cramping pains; dread of eating leads to major weight loss, and ischemic atrophy of the small bowel mucosa produces a spruelike syndrome. If advanced stenosis or occlusion of the superior mesenteric or celiac arteries, or both, can be shown angiographically, operation is advisable in most of these patients.

Asymptomatic patients in reasonably good health, having angiography for such lesions as renal cyst, and in whom advanced stenoses of two of the three major visceral arteries (celiac, superior mesenteric, and inferior mesenteric) are found incidentally are reasonable candidates for improvement in their visceral blood flow. Otherwise, a bout of hypotension from any cause might well lead to fatal intestinal necrosis. The salvage rate of patients with intestinal infarction is so very low that prophylactic arterial reconstruction seems justified, provided that stenosis is advanced.

When angiograms of the infrarenal aorta show an unusually large inferior mesenteric artery (e.g., 8 to 10 mm. in diameter), higher filming always shows significant lesions of the superior mesenteric and celiac vessels. Lateral films are vital to define these lesions.

CONTRAINDICATIONS

Noncritical stenoses, that is, anything less than 80 to 85% of the cross-sectional area of the arteries concerned.

PLANNING AND PREPARATION

In chronic abdominal pain syndromes, angiography often is done following the usual contrast studies of stomach, colon, kidney, and gallbladder. If any of these have been omitted, they should be carried out to reveal ancillary pathologic conditions requiring additional surgical attention.

Place a nasogastric tube preoperatively.

OPERATION

Position: Supine.

Incision: High midline or paramedian.

Perform a thorough abdominal exploration.

Aortomesenteric Bypass: For aortomesenteric bypass (Fig. 15-1) the first step in the exposure is to retract all of the small intestine to the patient's right. Elevate the transverse colon so that some tension is placed on the middle colic artery, which in turn imparts a tug to the superior mesenteric artery. In the left hand, grasp the entire mesentery of the small bowel, including the first loop of jejunum just below the ligament of Treitz, with the fingers on the patient's right and the thumb on the left. Through-and-through palpation at a depth just 1 or 2 cm. anterior to the aorta will usually detect the pulsation of an open superior mesenteric artery or the pencil-like cord of a sclerotic but pulseless vessel. Using the tip of the thumb as a guide, open the peritoneal coat of mesentery and identify the artery just distal to the middle colic branch. If, in a thick fatty mesentery, it is impossible to palpate the vessel, open the mesenteric peritoneum transversely and isolate the artery by patient blunt dissection, using any branch vessel as a guide.

Clear about 3 cm. of the artery; this may well include a branch or two.

Open the retroperitoneum over the anterior wall of the aorta halfway between the renal arteries and the inferior mesenteric and clear 5 cm. of aorta on each side, back to the lumbar branches.

Give 7500 units of heparin intravenously.

Inserting the Graft: Place a Satinsky or suitable vascular clamp on the aorta to exclude the entire vessel. Remove a 3 × 10 mm. full-thickness sliver from

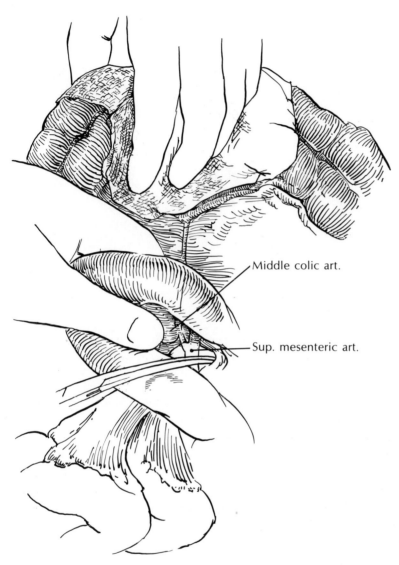

Middle colic art.

Sup. mesenteric art.

Figure 15-1.   Exposure of superior mesenteric artery.

the aortic wall in its long axis just to the right of the anterior midline. Place stay sutures at the edges of the aortotomy.

Cut an 8-mm. Dacron graft at a 45-degree angle, direct it upward, and suture it end to side into the aortotomy. Cut the upper end of the graft obliquely to fit against the left posterior wall of the superior mesenteric artery. This graft will be short (4 to 6 cm.).

Now place a curved vascular clamp, with the lock cephalad, from the left in a posterolateral direction onto the cleared segment of superior mesenteric artery.

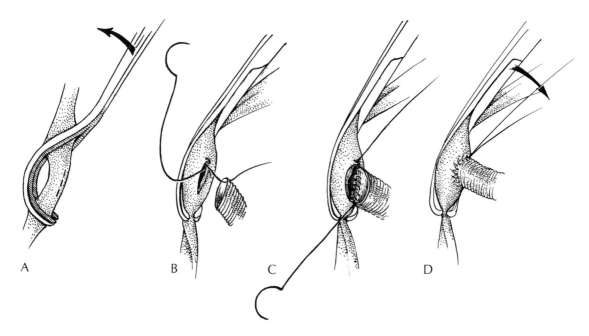

Figure 15-2.   (*A*) Superior mesenteric arteriotomy. (*B*) Beginning the anastomosis. (*C*) Posterior suture line. (*D*) Tying to suture of origin.

After rotating the artery 90 degrees by turning the handles of the clamp from left to right, make a 1-cm. arteriotomy (Fig. 15-2A).

A single suture attaches the uppermost angle of the graft to the superior end of the arteriotomy (Fig. 15-2B). Pass the needle back into the artery at a point 1 mm. posterior to that first stitch. Now the suture is inside the lumen. The posterior suture line is placed in an over-and-over manner from the inside until the lowermost angle is reached (Fig. 15-2C). The needle now comes outside the mesenteric artery, so that the completely accessible anterior suture line is run up from below as an everting over-and-over suture that is tied at the top angle of origin (Fig. 15-2D and 15-3).

To revascularize the celiac artery distribution (Fig. 15-4), bring an 8-mm. Dacron graft from the same aortic takeoff, or from the left side of an aortomesenteric graft, up to the inferior aspect of the splenic artery. Pass the graft through a tunnel created by blunt dissection through the mesocolon, posterior to the stomach and anterior to the pancreas, after the splenic artery is identified through a suitable opening in the gastrohepatic ligament. If the splenic artery is unduly small or atherosclerotic, the hepatic artery near its origin can be used.

Heparin neutralization by protamine sulfate may be desirable.

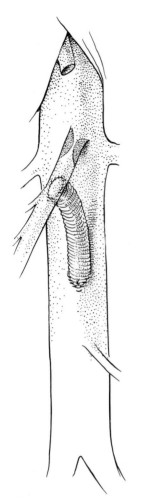

Figure 15-3. Aorta-to-superior mesenteric bypass completed.

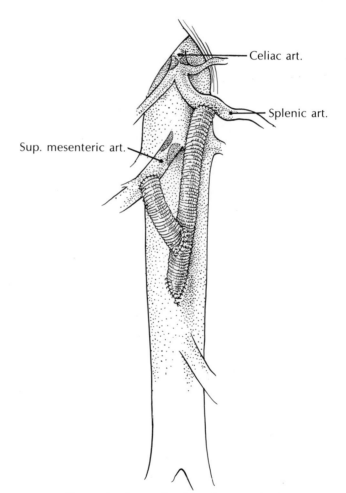

Celiac art.

Splenic art.

Sup. mesenteric art.

Figure 15-4. Combined aortosplenic and aortomesenteric bypass.

16   Lumbar sympathectomy

OBJECTIVES

To improve blood flow to the lower leg and foot by interruption of autonomic vasoconstrictor impulses to the vessels of the lower extremity.

Note: There is no thoracolumbar outflow from the spinal cord to the sympathetic chain below the third lumbar cord segment.

ANATOMIC RELATIONSHIPS

Autonomic impulses to the nerves of the lumbar and sacral plexuses from above L3 pass through white rami to the ganglionated chain, pass down the chain, and, via gray rami, join the somatic nerves for distribution (Fig. 16-1). Since no somatic nerve with a distribution lower than the femoral nerve is even partially initiated above L3, a complete denervation of the foot is accomplished by merely dividing the chain below the third lumbar ganglion. It is generally accepted, however, that there are opportunities for regeneration unless a certain arbitrary length of chain (about 2.5 cm.) is removed. Thus, in a patient requiring denervation of the foot only, the chain is divided below the third lumbar ganglion and resected for 2.5 cm. upward.

If denervation of the thigh or pelvic arteries, or both, is desired (and this is rare in modern practice), the connections between the sympathetic chain and the somatic nerves as high as the twelfth thoracic level must be interrupted. It is uncommon, but well recognized, that the twelfth thoracic nerve root can contribute autonomic efferents to the iliohypogastric, ilioinguinal, and genitofemoral combinations. However, in the majority of clinical situations in which high denervation is selected, the upper end of chain removal is set at just above the "first lumbar ganglion." This height of section is so dependable with respect to denervation of the iliofemoral arteries that routine removal of a twelfth or eleventh thoracic ganglion is not justified by the extent of the expected gain.

Identification of the ganglia by local appearance is difficult. Their size, the direction of rami, and the character of the sympathetic trunk are deceptive.

If one seeks orientation by the bony structures, the lower end of the chain division should be at or below the space between the bodies of the third and fourth lumbar vertebrae. The level of the upper division of chain, in order to be above the first lumbar ganglion in the rare patient in whom a high

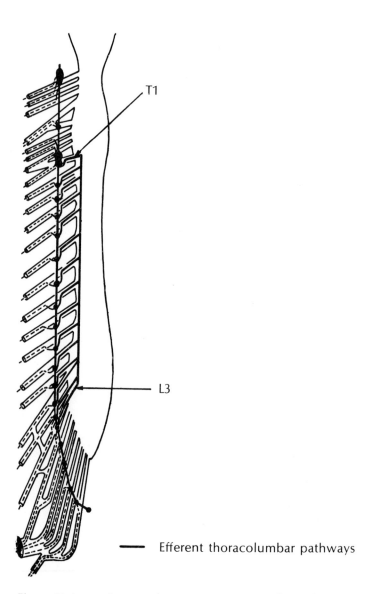

T1

L3

━━━ Efferent thoracolumbar pathways

Figure 16-1.   Autonomic nervous system. (Redrawn from J. C. White and R. H. Smithwick, *The Autonomic Nervous System* [3rd ed.]. New York: Macmillan, 1952.)

sympathectomy is planned, should be opposite the upper border of the first lumbar vertebra. These areas are identified by palpation of the twelfth rib, and thus by the twelfth vertebra from within (referring to the x-ray to be sure that no rib anomaly exists).

If one seeks orientation by the diaphragm, it is a nearly constant finding in the dissection of the chain that the muscular part of the crus must be divided for about 2 cm. in order to arrive opposite the upper border of the first lumbar vertebra, and thus above the first lumbar ganglion. Anomalous tendinous slips of the diaphragmatic crura must be disregarded. The chain usually becomes tenuous at the point where it is undergoing transition between the lumbar and thoracic regions and is coursing from the anterolateral to the lateral position in relation to the vertebral column. Often, no structure that looks like a ganglion is found in the crus of the diaphragm, although a sizable branch is usually encountered. For the purposes of this operative procedure, the junction of this branch with the sympathetic chain is then called the first lumbar ganglion.

INDICATIONS

These are limited by constraints that require further discussion. The increase in skin blood flow that follows lumbar sympathectomy is well demonstrated by the lasting increase in the skin temperature of the denervated foot. This effect on skin temperature is maximal when the arterial tree is anatomically normal but vasospasm is profound; it will be moderate when lower limb arteries are narrowed or obstructed at only one or two levels. There will be no effect on skin temperature at all when obliterative disease obstructs arterial flow at many levels and in many branch arteries. Significant increase in blood flow through femoropopliteal bypass grafts has been demonstrated by flowmeter studies to follow lumbar sympathectomy. This enhancement in flow is thought to result from the reduction in resistance of the arterial and arteriolar bed throughout the lower leg and foot.

It must be remembered that increases in blood flow to the foot resulting from sympathectomy are only small fractions of existing flow, whereas arterial reconstruction can multiply existing flow several times.

With vasospasm rare and multiple stenoses the rule, lumbar sympathectomy is seldom the treatment of choice for symptomatic obliterative arteriosclerosis. This operation cannot halt advancing necrosis or heal deep gangrene over the foot. It rarely brings relief when rest pain is constant and rubor is striking. It will not improve diabetic neuritis or lower the level of amputation.

Whereas restoration of mainstem arterial flow by reconstruction will cure intermittent claudication, sympathectomy will increase walking distance by perhaps 15 or 20%. Lumbar sympathectomy has no place in acute arterial occlusions causing marked ischemia. In advanced diabetic neuropathy, the dorsolateral columns of the lumbar cord giving rise to the sympathetic white rami show sufficient degeneration to produce an autosympathectomy effect.

Lumbar sympathectomy in arteriosclerotic obliterative disease is best considered when a palpable popliteal pulse rules out reconstruction, deterioration of the limb is slow, infection is absent, and any necrosis is stable, superficial, and limited to one or two toes or the heel.

Specific Indications: These are as follows.

1. Unusual cases of obliterative arteriosclerosis, as described.
2. Old traumatic mainstem arterial interruption not susceptible to reconstruction.
3. Raynaud's disease (rare in the feet).
4. Established secondary Raynaud's phenomena (such as in Buerger's disease).
5. Sensitivity to cold following cold injury.
6. Hyperhidrosis.
7. True causalgia.
8. In aortoiliac reconstruction, when the femoral arteries are also obstructed (see Chap. 3).

CONTRAINDICATIONS

1. In arteriosclerosis obliterans with rest pain, gangrene that is other than superficial, very local, and stable.
2. Acute arterial occlusion.
3. After-cold injury, with chronic pain or edema and no cold sensitivity.
4. Post-traumatic pain syndromes of the lower extremity, except for true causalgia.
5. Amputation stump or phantom pain.
6. Venous or lymphatic stasis.

PLANNING AND PREPARATION

In cases of arteriosclerosis and absent popliteal pulses, make arteriograms to determine the patient's suitability for the preferred treatment of arterial reconstruction.

Because of the slow appearance of benefit after sympathectomy in organic obliterative arterial disease, observation for a skin temperature rise after temporary lumbar sympathetic nerve block is of little prognostic use in arteriosclerosis. For causalgia and for many of the vasospasms, however, it is a required preliminary maneuver to assess the potential value of sympathectomy.

The goal of the operation is to remove at least two, and preferably three, of the four lumbar sympathetic ganglia as they are found between the proximal common iliac vessels and the diaphragmatic crura. In males it is desirable to leave the first lumbar ganglion in place so that ejaculation will not be affected. Moreover, the sympathetic denervation of the lower leg and foot that follows resection of the second and third lumbar ganglia may well accomplish the central objective without added denervation of the iliac vessel. By making certain that the first ganglion removed lies beneath the right common iliac vein or the left common iliac artery, that no more than three are removed, and that the cephalad dissection stops short of the crus of the diaphragm, L1 can be preserved. The opportunities for regeneration are less, and the elimination of crossover connections from the opposite side are greater, if a minimum of two ganglia including 2.5 cm. of chain (or preferably three ganglia) are removed.

Two approaches are described.

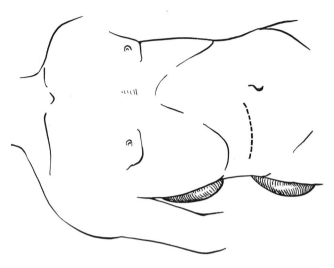

Figure 16-2.   Incision. (Modified from F. J. Veith, D. C. Marshall, and C. Crane, *Surg. Gynecol. Obstet.* 119:109, 1964.)

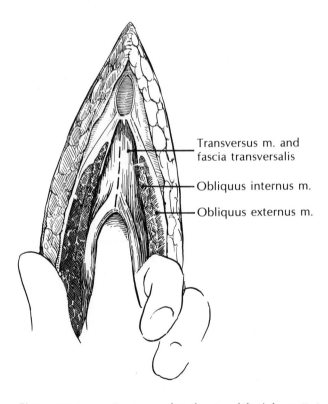

Transversus m. and fascia transversalis

Obliquus internus m.

Obliquus externus m.

Figure 16-3.   Exposure details. (Modified from F. J. Veith, D. C. Marshall, and C. Crane, *Surg. Gynecol. Obstet.* 119:109, 1964.)

APPROACH 1: ANTERIOR TRANSVERSE INCISION

Position: Supine, side of operation held up 20 degrees by sandbags under the thorax and hip.

Incision and Exposure: Start the skin incision 2 cm. above and 6 cm. lateral to the umbilicus and carry it directly laterally for 10 cm. to the anterior axillary line (Fig. 16-2). The external and internal oblique muscles, their aponeuroses, and the anterior rectus sheath are divided in line with the skin incision (Fig. 16-3). The lateral 4 cm. of the rectus muscle is divided. The transversus abdominis muscle is split in the direction of its fibers, and the fascia transversalis is opened at the most lateral aspect of the incision. Here, properitoneal fat tends to separate this layer from the peritoneum.

  Dissect the peritoneum free medially with the index finger before extending the incision in the fascia transversalis (Fig. 16-4). With clamps on the fascia transversalis, the peritoneum is further dissected free in all directions while the posterior rectus sheath is finally opened to the limit of the skin incision.

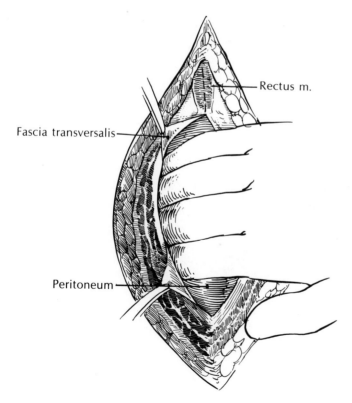

Rectus m.

Fascia transversalis

Peritoneum

Figure 16-4.   Exposure details. (Modified from F. J. Veith, D. C. Marshall, and C. Crane, *Surg. Gynecol. Obstet.* 119:109, 1964.)

Place a moist gauze pad and a 2-inch Deaver retractor over the peritoneal sac while the plane just anterior to the psoas muscle is entered and developed medially to the vena cava on the right side. Place a second deep retractor superiorly to hold back the fatty tissue (Fig. 16-5).

With the vena cava gently retracted forward and medially, the midlumbar vertebrae are palpated directly posteromedial to the vena cava. A layer of fatty areolar tissue overlying the groove between the psoas muscle and the vena cava is opened, and the anterolateral aspect of the vertebral bodies lying just above the right common iliac vein is exposed. Firm palpation with the index finger over these vertebrae in the coronal plane will reveal the slippery, firm cord that is the lumbar sympathetic chain or the ovoid swelling of a ganglion.

Removal of Sympathetic Chain: With a nerve hook under the chain, follow it in both directions, looking for confirming rami and ganglia (Fig. 16-6). The chain may lie beneath a lumbar artery or vein. In this case it is sometimes easier to divide the chain and pull it out from underneath such a vessel than to dissect and divide the vessel itself.

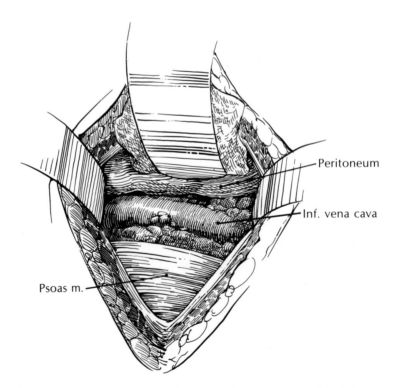

Figure 16-5.   Exposure of paravertebral area. (Modified from F. J. Veith, D. C. Marshall, and C. Crane, *Surg. Gynecol. Obstet.* 119:109, 1964.)

Work downward first, dividing rami and freeing the chain of fascial strands. Under the common iliac vein on the right or the iliac artery on the left, apply a clip and divide below a well-defined ganglion. Catch the lower end of the chain in a right-angled clamp to put mild tension on it downward and away from the spine; this makes further dissection upward much easier. After repeated replacement of gauze pads and retractors, another ganglion or so and another 2.5 cm. of chain can be obtained superiorly just before the

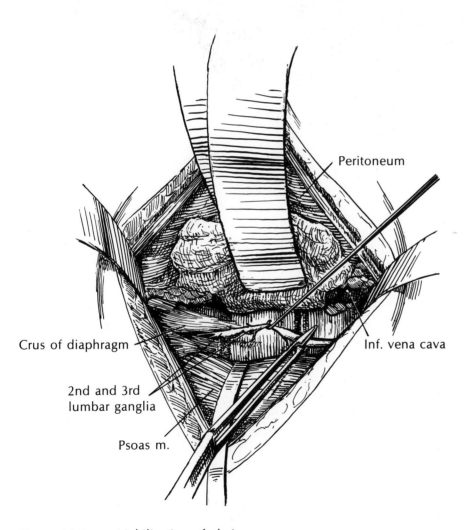

Peritoneum

Crus of diaphragm

Inf. vena cava

2nd and 3rd
lumbar ganglia

Psoas m.

Figure 16-6.   Mobilization of chain.

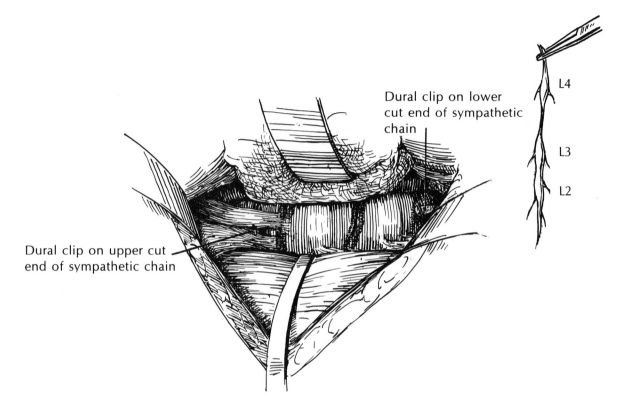

Dural clip on lower
cut end of sympathetic
chain

Dural clip on upper cut
end of sympathetic chain

L4

L3

L2

Figure 16-7.   Removal of chain.

thinning chain disappears into the muscle of the diaphragmatic crus. Apply a clip at this point, which is below L1 and above L2. Remove 7 to 10 cm. of chain (Fig. 16-7). If there is any doubt, it is good to confirm the identity of the tissue by immediate frozen section.

Hemostasis should be perfect before closure is begun.

It is most important to close the posterior rectus sheath and the fascia transversalis very carefully in one continuous layer to the full lateral extent of the incision, using chromic catgut. The internal oblique aponeurosis and accompanying muscle are also closed with running chromic catgut. The anterior rectus sheath and the aponeurosis of the external oblique are closed with interrupted silk.

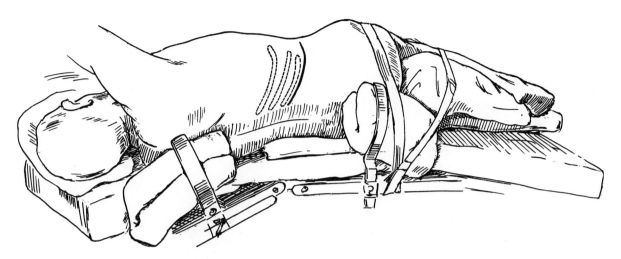

Figure 16-8.   Position and incision.

APPROACH 2: POSTERIOR LOIN INCISION

This approach, which was preferred by Smithwick,* has these advantages: (1) it cuts across less muscle, (2) it requires less retraction of the vena cava, and (3) in the right-sided operation, it provides somewhat better visualization of the diaphragmatic crus and of the first lumbar ganglion than do anterior approaches. Its disadvantages are that it requires perfect positioning of the patient and that the position tends to decrease venous return via the vena cava. Further, the incision is small and does not allow visualization by the assistants or easy freer access for repairing deep structures in case of inadvertent injury. It is now used only in those rare instances in which removal of L1 is indicated and by those who are familiar with the approach.

Position: Lateral, strongly flexed at the waist, tilted 20 degrees toward the supine, upper thigh flexed to relax the psoas muscle, careful protection of the feet, pillow between the legs.

Incision and Exposure: Start the skin incision 2 cm. from the outer edge of the sacrospinalis muscle and 2 cm. below the lower border of the twelfth rib. Carry it parallel to the twelfth rib until its tip is reached and thence transversely for a total length of 15 cm. (Fig. 16-8).

*J. C. White, R. H. Smithwick, and F. A. Simeone. *The Autonomic Nervous System* (3rd ed.). New York: Macmillan, 1952.

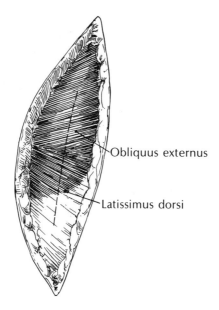

Figure 16-9.   Incision details.

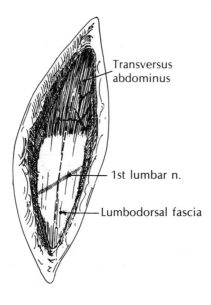

Figure 16-10.   Incision details.

The first assistant stands on the same side as the surgeon.

Divide the muscles, using the lumbar trigone (Petit's triangle) as a guide for the center of muscle incision (Fig. 16-9). Preserve the nerves (Fig. 16-10). Develop the retroperitoneal area by finger and scissors dissection. Palpate the chain.

Insert a dry pack in toto. Use a deep S-shaped retractor against the peritoneum and a spatula on the psoas muscle.

Incise the prevertebral fascia over the sympathetic chain. Elevate the chain with a nerve hook. The first assistant controls the changing positions of the S-shaped retractor and the psoas muscle retractor.

Dissection: Dissect and remove the chain as in Approach 1. When removing L1, divide that part of the muscle of the diaphragmatic crus that lies lateral to the chain, which will then be seen as a thin strand ascending and coursing slightly laterally, until the small ganglion, or more commonly the branch described on page 155, comes into view. This will usually be 2 cm. above L2.

Close with silk to the lumbodorsal fascia, intermuscular fasciae, deep fascia of the back, and skin, using small bites and avoiding wide muscle sutures.

POSTOPERATIVE MANAGEMENT

Take x-ray films of the lumbar and lower dorsal spines for identification of marking clips to document the level of chain removal.

Genitofemoral, ilioinguinal, or other neuritis associated with the roots of the first and second lumbar nerves is very common, regardless of the type of operative approach or the handling. It will always disappear but may take weeks or months. The only treatment is reassurance.

17 Transaxillary dorsal sympathectomy

THE FIRST THORACIC and inferior cervical ganglia fuse to form the stellate (cervicothoracic) ganglion, which has diffuse connections with the spinal nerves. Connections between the second and third thoracic ganglia and the brachial plexus can occur without the fibers' passing through the first thoracic ganglion. In a radical sympathectomy, the sympathetic chain containing the stellate ganglion and the second, third, fourth, and fifth ganglia is removed, and the second and third thoracic nerves and their roots for 3 cm. outside the vertebral column, starting intraspinally, are resected. Following this operation, laboratory evidence of persistent or recurrent sympathetic innervation will be absent in over 70% of patients and any clinical evidence will be lacking in nearly all of them. Its telling disadvantage is the possible creation of Horner's syndrome, which is disfiguring and subjectively annoying.

OBJECTIVES

The objective of radical sympathectomy in the majority of patients is to interrupt the autonomic efferent impulses to the vessels of the upper extremity without inducing a frank Horner's syndrome. This is best done by a somewhat limited sympathectomy consisting of resection of the chain through the center of the stellate ganglion, between the inferior cervical and the first thoracic ganglia, and removing the first three dorsal ganglia. The spinal nerves are left intact. Following this operation, laboratory evidence of recurrence of some sympathetic function will be observed in all but a very few patients, but the operation will give clinical satisfaction in about 75% of patients.

INDICATIONS

Hyperhidrosis interfering with work.
Raynaud's disease when fingertip ulceration or pain is present.
Selected cases of causalgia, late frostbite, and scleroderma.

CONTRAINDICATIONS

Lesser vasospasms without tissue change or disability.
Apical lung or pleural disease.

167

PLANNING AND PREPARATION

The patient should understand that a full Horner's syndrome is a remote possibility and that a chest tube may be in place for a few days.

OPERATION

Position: Lateral decubitus, with the side to be operated on uppermost (Fig. 17-1). The position of the arm is critical. The upper arm is abducted to 100 degrees, with the elbow flexed to a right angle and the forearm, well-padded, carefully bound to a malleable overhead frame. To avoid stretch injury to the brachial plexus it is important that the arm not be further abducted.

Incision and Exposure: Directly over the second interspace. Incision length is limited by the pectoralis major muscle anteriorly and the latissimus dorsi muscle posteriorly.

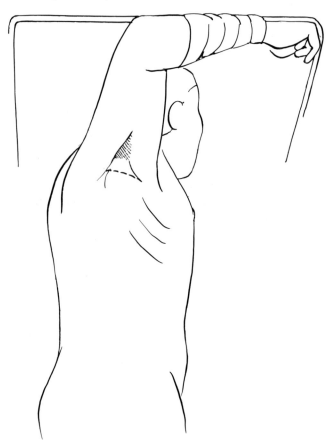

Figure 17-1.   Position and incision.

As the 8-cm. incision is deepened through the axillary fat and the deep fascia is opened, avoid the thoracodorsal and long thoracic nerves. Place retractors on each of these muscles to widen the distance between them.

Split the serratus anterior muscle in the direction of its fibers and divide the intercostal muscles of the second interspace with the scalpel until the pleura is exposed (Fig. 17-2).

After the pleura is opened and the rib spreader placed, open this retractor *very slowly* over 5 minutes. This greatly reduces postoperative pain and the likelihood of rib fracture (Fig. 17-3).

Place a moist gauze pad over the apex of the lung, which is collapsed downward under a deep Deaver or heart-shaped retractor.

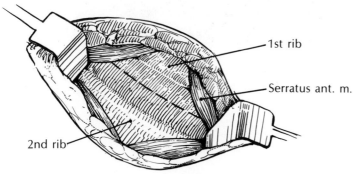

Figure 17-2.   Division of intercostal muscle.

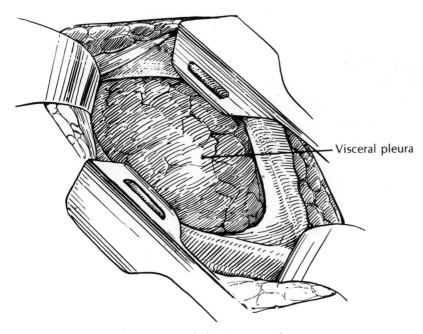

Figure 17-3.   Pleura opened, lung exposed.

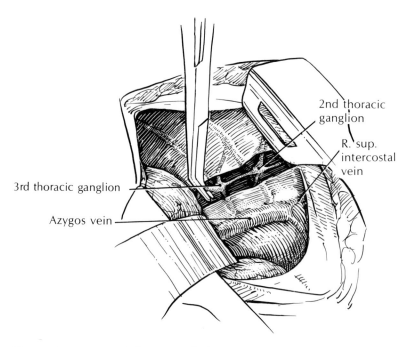

Figure 17-4.   Mobilization of chain.

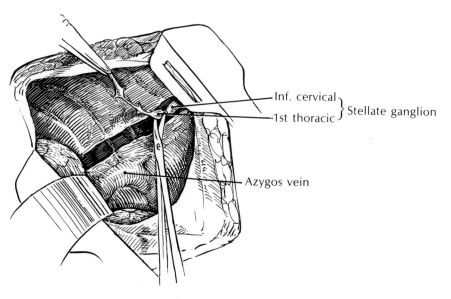

Figure 17-5.   Division of chain below the inferior cervical ganglion.

An intrathoracic light source on either a retractor or a long Lucite carrier is vital. On the right, the sympathetic chain will be seen beneath the parietal pleural lying on the heads of the ribs just 3 cm. or so lateral to the right superior intercostal and azygos veins. On the left, the chain lies just lateral to the aorta.

Finally, establish the identity of the first rib by proving the absence of any rib above it. Gentle palpation of the thoracic outlet with a long instrument such as a full-length clamp will completely clarify which is the first rib.

Identify the stellate ganglion by its dumbbell shape. The lower half, the first thoracic ganglion, lies just below and on the inferior border of the first rib, while the upper half lies on the head of this rib.

Dissection: Open the pleura with a long-handled knife directly over the chain and just below the fourth ganglion (Fig. 17-4). The tips of a long right-angled clamp are used for elevation and blunt dissection of the pleura in a cephalad direction. Control any bleeding at once by electrocoagulation combined with pressure and packing. Remove the first, second, and third thoracic ganglia (Fig. 17-5) from below upward.

Hemostasis should be very careful and complete, as hemothorax is the most common complication of this procedure.

If there is uncontrolled oozing, or if many adhesions have been divided, place a chest tube for underwater seal. Although this is rarely necessary, it is better to use it when in doubt.

No attempt is made to close either pleural layer. After full expansion of the lung, close the deep fascia with continuous chromic catgut. Interrupted sutures approximate the subcutaneous tissue, and a continuous plastic skin suture is used.

Obtain a chest film on the day after operation—sooner, of course, if unexpected chest symptoms or signs should appear.

18 Notes on nonoperative treatment of venous stasis

PHYSIOLOGIC PRINCIPLES

The venous pressure in the lower extremities of a person who is standing quietly is equal to the hydrostatic pressure of the column of blood between the area concerned and the heart, whether the veins are incompetent or normal. This pressure is higher than can be continuously tolerated by the tissues of the lower leg. Trouble is avoided in the normal leg by contraction of the muscles, which repeatedly lowers the venous pressure to tolerable levels if the valves of the deep veins of the calf are functioning normally. This does not occur when the valves are incompetent, as in the postphlebitic state. Thus "elevated venous pressure" in the extremity of a person with abnormal veins means a standing pressure that cannot be lowered by walking. The therapeutic implications of these principles have resulted in two methods of bringing about normal local venous pressure and one method of combating the effects of abnormal pressures:

1. Surgical elimination of the incompetent veins, which allows pressure to be brought down by the normal mechanism of walking. The efficacy of this procedure depends upon the number of normal veins remaining afterward. It is thus curative in most patients with primary varicose veins in whom the deep veins are normal, but far less effective in those whose deep veins have been damaged by previous phlebitis.
2. Elevation of the legs, which decreases pressure by removing the hydrostatic element.
3. External elastic support. The steep gradient across the capillary wall between increased capillary pressure and tissue pressure can be eliminated by increasing the tissue pressure. This is effected by firmly wrapping the leg in an elastic bandage.

NONOPERATIVE MANAGEMENT

Although the following principles may be helpful in the management of venous stasis from any cause, they are primarily directed to the postphlebitic state. It is the rare patient whose edema or ulcer cannot be controlled by a combination of nonoperative measures, namely, elevation and elastic support.

Elevation of Legs: A patient who is employed has difficulty finding time to elevate his legs during the working day. However, he should attempt to lie with his legs elevated for half an hour in the middle of the day. It is good for him to place 3-inch blocks under the foot of his bed in order to allow complete drainage of edema fluid by morning.

The patient who is not working regularly outside the home can arrange to lie down more often, perhaps every 3 hours. Many housewives without small children around the house can do this. Patients who have had recent iliofemoral phlebitis should be taught the importance of avoiding edema during the first six months after onset, when venous collaterals are developing. They should get off their feet as frequently as is necessary to accomplish this during this period.

Elastic Support: The following types of elastic support are available:

1. Elastic cotton wrap-around bandages.
2. Rubberized elastic wrap-around bandages.
3. Elastic stockings. *Note:* These should rarely extend above the knee, should stretch both ways, and may be heavy or light, depending on the degree of edema.
4. Elastic adhesive.
5. Elastic bandage lined with foam rubber.
6. Unna's paste boot.
7. Inflatable legging.

The choice in a patient with chronic edema usually lies between a rubberized wrap-around bandage and an elastic stocking. Teach the patient to use the bandage at the outset, since when he learns he can apply it more effectively than anyone else. Although many patients will later change to a stocking, others will wish to retain the wrap-around bandage (Fig. 18-1). Its advantages are that it can always be applied with appropriate pressure and that pads and dressings can be used under it. Its disadvantages are that it becomes disarranged easily and that it is more unsightly than a stocking.

The elastic bandage with incorporated foam rubber and the inflatable legging are used for more advanced and recalcitrant cases and thus are not in competition with the above methods.

Support should be applied before arising in the morning, when swelling has

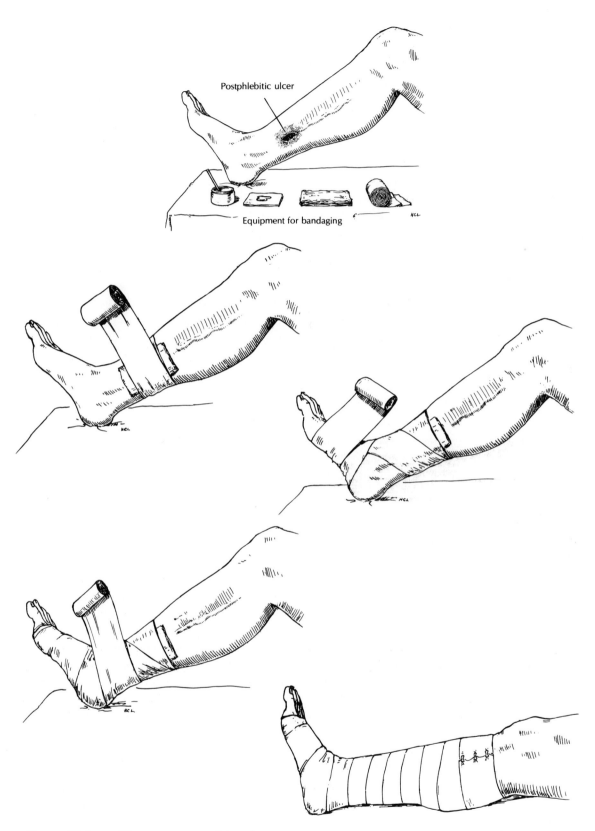

Postphlebitic ulcer

Equipment for bandaging

Figure 18-1. The wrap-around bandage.

not had a chance to appear. It should go from the base of the toes to below the knee and include the heel.

Unna's paste boot* or the elastic adhesive are used more often in patients with open ulceration or dermatitis. The former comes prepared under various trade names. The elastic adhesive is applied over a cotton bandage in order to make some provision for absorption of exudate and to keep the adhesive off the skin. It can also be applied over a paste boot. It is left on for one to two weeks, depending on the degree of ulceration and exudation beneath it. Carefully avoid tight wrapping in patients with arterial insufficiency.

Treat ulcers that require more frequent examination by appropriate local care and dress with a gauze sponge supported with a pressure pad of Cellucotton, which can simultaneously provide spongy pressure and absorb exudate. Apply the wrap-around elastic bandage over this pad.

Treatment of Ulcers and Dermatitis: Ulcers that are superficially infected are treated by an appropriate ointment and elastic support as outlined. Daily cleansing with soap and water is important.

If the ulcer is surrounded by infection, put the patient to bed with the leg elevated for a few days and apply wet dressings.

Patients whose ulcers are painful often use ointments with phenol in them. This may cause tissue damage and should be forbidden. The patient should remain in bed for healing if feasible.

Dermatitis without ulcer may not respond to ointments and may become worse on wetting or under paste casts. Here, bed rest and elevation are generally necessary. A weak alcoholic lotion (such as witch hazel) often helps as an adjunct.

Education and Weight Control: Make certain that the patient with unrelieved venous incompetence understands the importance of weight control and the specific dietary measures that will achieve and maintain it.

It is the physician's responsibility to see that his patient can put on his own elastic support properly and can apply the necessary local dressing correctly.

Too often, surgeons who best understand the principles underlying these measures are least willing to devote the necessary time to educating their patients. The instruction takes patience but will be rewarding in terms of minimizing the total time involved in patient care and will greatly decrease the patient's disability.

---

*Unna, whom some have called the father of modern dermatology, first used a medicated boot for stasis ulcers. His paste contained zinc oxide, glycerin, and mucilage of acacia. Many packaged bandages have succeeded the paste. They still contain zinc oxide and glycerin, the physical properties of the medicament being more important than the chemical properties.

19 *Stripping of long and short saphenous veins*

OBJECTIVES

To remove the main channels carrying blood to varicose veins.

To remove potential new channels that could form to feed the varices after the main ones have been destroyed.

INDICATIONS

Tortuous, dilated veins and either fatigue on standing, discomfort in the veins themselves, or stasis pigmentation, dermatitis, or ulcer.

CONTRAINDICATIONS

Postphlebitic syndrome in the absence of a dilated saphenous trunk.

PLANNING AND PREPARATION

If ulcer or dermatitis is present, a suitable preliminary period of bed rest and limb elevation is indicated.

Tests for venous function should be performed.

Trendelenberg's or Perthes' test should be performed on all patients with varicose veins to determine (1) whether or not the deep and communicating veins (which should, for this purpose, be considered part of the deep system) are competent and (2) which elements of the skin veins (the long saphenous, the accessory saphenous, the short saphenous, or an unusual communicating vein) are feeding the varices.

Trendelenberg's test is performed using a firm band applied below the knee after the leg has been sharply elevated and the veins emptied. The patient then stands, and the veins are observed for the time of maximum filling, which normally occurs after a lapse of over 30 seconds while the band is in place. If total filling occurs before that time, it can be assumed that the deep system is incompetent. If filling occurs after 30 seconds, the test should be repeated with the tourniquet applied at varying levels, proceeding upward to determine the level of the communicating vein that is feeding the varices. Release of the tourniquet at the end of the test period will determine whether or not the veins fill additionally by retrograde flow downward, giving added proof, if any is needed, that they are incompetent.

Perthes' test is an appraisal of the ability of the patient's deep and communicating veins, aided by the pump action of the calf muscles during walking, to move blood out of the dilated skin veins into the deep veins and upward. A band is applied at knee level while the patient is upright, and the varicose veins below this level are observed for emptying or decrease in pressure during walking.

Venography to determine disease of the deep system is performed only when these tests are inconclusive.

The course of the main saphenous trunk is marked the night before operation with two or three cutaneous needle scratches, which are designed to identify the place on the skin at which an extra incision must be made in case the initial stripping does not remove the entire main vein. Any communicating vein that arises at a point other than along the course of the main trunk should be marked. Do not mark large clusters of varices or tortuous veins, since these cannot be stripped and, at the initial operation at least, should not be excised.

Palpable long saphenous, accessory saphenous, and short saphenous veins are searched for. The patient must stand for at least 5 minutes before marking is done in order to distend the veins properly.

The whole lower extremity, groin, and lower abdomen are shaved, pedicure is performed, and the whole body is cleansed, particularly the foot areas, with a bath the night before or on the morning of operation.

The best plan is to remove the long and short saphenous veins from each extremity in which operation is indicated. The accessory saphenous vein is also to be removed if it has been identified preoperatively or is found at operation. It is not to be hunted for if not percussible preoperatively or seen in the femoral wound at operation.

If both lower extremities have long saphenous varices and short saphenous veins are not contributing to them, it is better to do bilateral long saphenous vein stripping and leave the short saphenous vein stripping for a later operation. A bilateral long and short saphenous vein stripping at one sitting is too cumbersome and time-consuming, because of the need for position change and redraping, to make it advisable as a routine.

PROCEDURE

Position and Draping: Supine. Legs elevated at a 20-degree angle for hemostasis.

Prepare the skin from the umbilicus to the base of the toes, including the pubis.

Place a glove over the forefoot. Use a laparotomy sheet with a hole in it to put the leg through.

Incision: Make the first incision anterior to and below the medial malleolus, parallel to and just above the shoe line, just long enough to admit a stripper (Fig. 19-1).

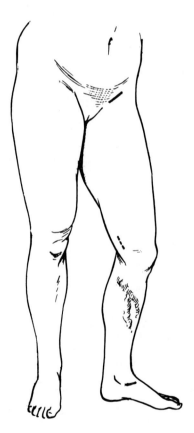

Figure 19-1.   Incisions.

Stripping: Insert the stripper into the divided long saphenous vein and pass it to the femoral triangle (Fig. 19-2).

Make a 3-cm. incision centering over the stripper in the crease of the groin. Identify the vein with the stripper in it and divide it.

Strip the vein out through the groin incision, having secured the vein to the stripper at the ankle with a heavy ligature (Fig. 19-3). This maneuver is accomplished by a steady pull on the stripper while an assistant breaks the branches by pulling on the tensed skin with gauze (Fig. 19-4).

Apply pressure for 2 to 3 minutes over the stripped tunnel to procure hemostasis. An alternative method is to wrap a sterile elastic bandage from the toes upward as the stripper is withdrawn.

Examine the specimen to see that the whole length of vein has been removed (Fig. 19-5). If part of the specimen shows only one wall of the vein, do nothing further. If a stripper with an end too small for the diameter of the vein has been used and the vein has invaginated and broken, make a small incision, using one of the preoperative scratch marks as a guide, in order to recover it. Then attempt further stripping. An external stripper may be useful under these circumstances.

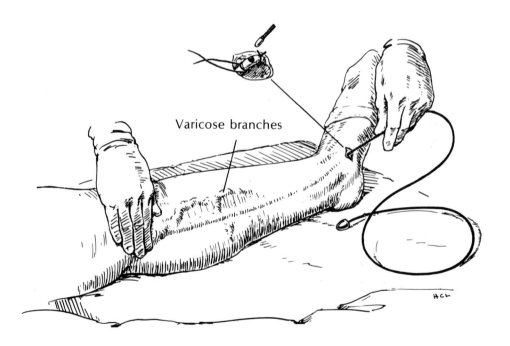

Figure 19-2.   Stripper insertion.

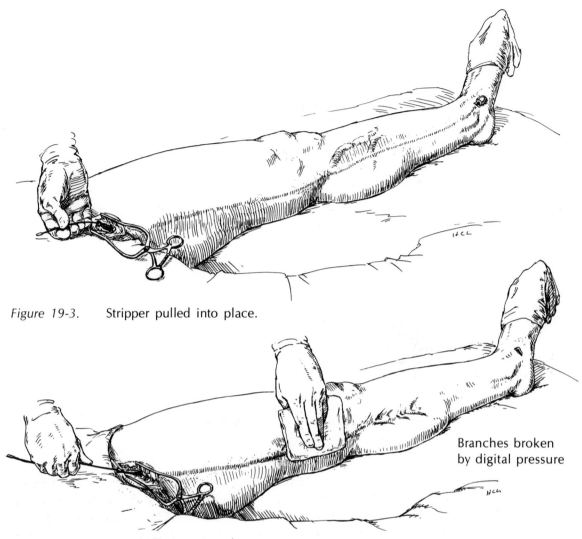

Figure 19-3.   Stripper pulled into place.

Branches broken
by digital pressure

Figure 19-4.   Vein halfway stripped out.

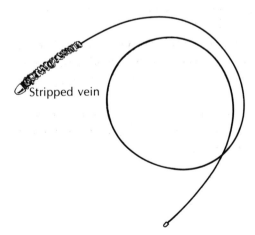

Stripped vein

Figure 19-5.   Stripper out with vein telescoped upon it.

Superf. epigastric vein   Superf. circumflex iliac
                                       art. and
Saphenous   vein
    vein
Superf. ext.
pudendal vein

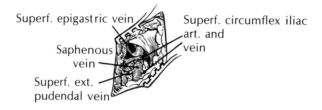

Figure 19-6.   Saphenofemoral dissection. For clarity, relationships are shown before stripping.

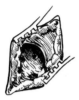

Figure 19-7.   Saphenous vein ligated and divided.

Dissect the proximal stump of the vein (Fig. 19-6). Divide all branches between the level of the division and the femoral vein. Identify the level of the femoral vein by palpation of the artery which will be a guide to the depth of the dissection. Excise the vein and ligate the stump at the femoral vein (Fig. 19-7).

Strip the short saphenous vein, inserting the stripper via a short longitudinal incision behind the lateral malleolus and withdrawing it through a transverse incision in the popliteal space (Fig. 19-8).

Knead all blood clot out of the stripped subcutaneous tunnels. External pressure over the tunnels is not necessary unless bleeding continues. Expression of clot is the most important factor in preventing postoperative hematoma and ecchymosis.

Close all wounds below the knee with fine sutures. This is important in rendering the incision less conspicuous in women. Close the remaining wounds with silk or other routine suture material.

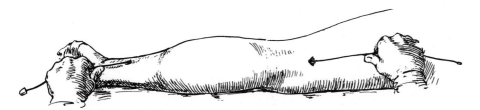

Figure 19-8.   Short saphenous vein stripping.

POSTOPERATIVE MANAGEMENT

Use an elastic bandage extending from the toes to below the knees (Fig. 19-9). It is not necessary above the knee except in the rare cases in which bleeding has been a problem.

Elevate the foot of the bed on 3-inch blocks. After the effects of the anesthetic have worn off, the patient may stand and walk provided firm elastic support of the lower leg is maintained. Although dependency should be limited on the day of operation, it may be allowed in patients who had limited operations; in these simple cases the operation may be considered "ambulatory surgery." For three or four days it is good to avoid continuous or prolonged dependency. However, full activity during the period of dependency is permitted. Maintain elastic support until suture removal on the seventh or eighth day.

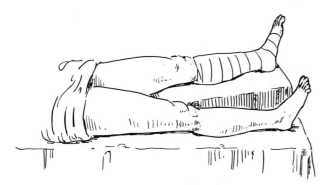

Figure 19-9.   Postoperative bandage.

Comment: For patients suffering from postphlebitic syndrome, the length of convalescence depends on such factors as the degree of dermatitis and edema. In these patients, saphenous stripping is only one of several maneuvers in rehabilitation.

Injections of sclerosing material may be necessary later. In general, injections should not be given without previous stripping or ligation, or the veins will soon recanalize. The only exception to this rule is a small varix that a woman wishes ablated for cosmetic reasons only.

In recurrent cases, or in patients who have had multiple previous injections, the veins must be removed by excision through a long incision in the calf. In so doing, flaps no wider than 4 cm. each should be elevated and the veins superficial to the deep fascia removed. This is not a subfascial "ligation of communicators," but a method of removing the skin veins when they are not amenable to stripping.

20 Excision and graft of stasis ulcer and ligation of communicating veins

OBJECTIVES

To remove an area of skin and fascia so damaged that it cannot heal properly. Following application of the new skin, the patient has a better opportunity to respond to a conservative regimen.

To interrupt the communicating veins, which are the channels causing high-pressure venous blood to pool in the diseased area.

INDICATIONS

In most cases appropriate stripping or excision of varicose veins, as outlined in Chapter 19, has been done previously if indicated. If not, it should be done before deciding on an excision and graft. If the patient has postphlebitic syndrome and no readily apparent varicosities, vein stripping alone cannot be counted on to cure the ulcer. Excision and graft or ligation of communicating veins, or both, are then done at the outset, with stripping of the long saphenous vein made part of the same procedure.

Ulceration uncontrolled by these surgical procedures, and a strict regimen of regulated dependency and elastic support is, then, the chief indication; patients vary widely in their ability to carry out such a regimen. Operation is undertaken earlier on those who have neither the interest, intellect, nor leisure to adhere to the regimen, but since it is also necessary postoperatively, an operation should be done only after an extended trial of nonoperative management and education of the patient in self-care.

CONTRAINDICATIONS

Edema without ulceration.
  Pigmentation or dermatitis only.

PLANNING AND PREPARATION

Before operation, enforce bed rest with elevation of the leg and application of wet dressings for as long as is necessary to reach maximum improvement in the ulcer and surrounding tissues. By this means, healing can be induced in many patients.

Culture the ulcer for isolation of organisms and determination of their sensitivity to antibiotics.

OPERATION

Apply a double amount of the usual skin preparation.

Position: Supine. Elevate the foot of the table to a 20-degree angle.

Incision: Outline the area to be excised by determining where the skin and subcutaneous tissues are soft. The incision can rarely be made outside the area of pigmentation (Fig. 20-1).

Dissection: Carry the posterior part of the incision down through the deep fascia and remove the whole skin and fascial segment from posterior to anterior, staying between the deep fascia superficially and the periosteum and tendon sheaths deeply. The anterior part of the skin incision is made as one proceeds. Beware of dissection deep to the Achilles tendon. The saphenous nerve is divided in the process, but this causes little disability.

The communicating veins are found on a longitudinal line extending from the posterior aspect of the medial malleolus (Fig. 20-2). Extend this incision to mid-calf.

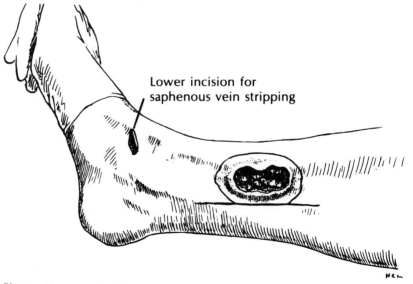

Lower incision for
saphenous vein stripping

Figure 20-1.   Incisions.

Apply a split-thickness graft taken from the thigh of the same leg (Fig. 20-3).

Apply an appropriate pressure dressing. An excellent one consists of fine-meshed gauze covered with coarse-mesh gauze, with cotton waste on top, the whole being held in place with sutures. Use plaster casing or a splint from the toes to the mid-thigh to immobilize the ankle joint.

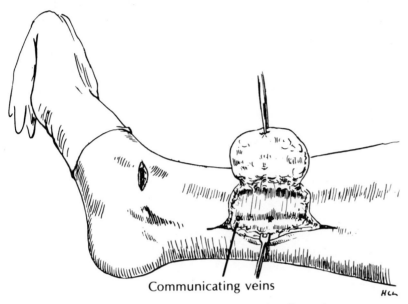

Communicating veins

Figure 20-2.   Excision, communicating veins ligated.

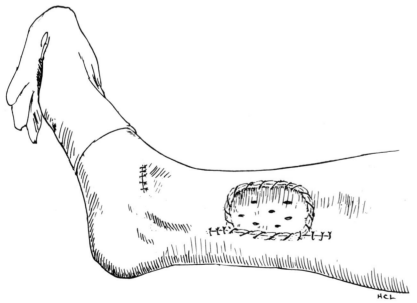

Figure 20-3.   Closure with split-thickness graft.

POSTOPERATIVE MANAGEMENT

Elevate the leg continuously.

Change the dressing first on the fifth day; care of the graft following this is subject to individual preference. A good approach is to leave the area exposed to the open air under a protective cocoon. This provides an opportunity to employ wet dressings to areas that have not taken. Dependency of the foot must be on a very slowly graduated schedule (e.g., 5 minutes per hour at first) and always accompanied by local pressure on the grafted area with elastic support of the whole leg. Even in the best of circumstances, return to the preoperative schedule of ambulation is not possible for two to three weeks.

21 Diagnosis and management of thromboembolism

In about 50% of instances, deep venous thrombosis and pulmonary embolism are clinically silent.

Deep venous thrombosis as much as seven to ten days old when first diagnosed rarely causes pulmonary embolism.

A normal lung scan is certain evidence that recent embolism has not occurred.

An abnormal lung scan following a clear chest film gives almost perfect evidence for pulmonary embolism. The rare exceptions are caused by emphysematous blebs.

A negative pulmonary arteriogram is certain evidence that no embolus larger than 5 to 6 mm. has lodged in the pulmonary arterial tree.

Central pulmonary embolism occluding less than 50% of the cross-sectional area of the pulmonary artery may be entirely silent except for minimal dyspnea and tachycardia, often overlooked.

For pulmonary embolism to cause hypotension in patients with essentially normal cardiopulmonary function, more than 50% of the cross-sectional area of the pulmonary arterial distribution must be occluded. Under these circumstances the mean pulmonary artery pressure will exceed 25 mm Hg, and acute cor pulmonale will result.

Pleuritic chest pain, hemoptysis, pleural fluid accumulation, a parenchymal infiltrate, and fever due to pulmonary embolism are all evidence of pulmonary infarction from thrombus that lodged 24 to 48 hours earlier.

Pleural fluid caused by pulmonary embolism is more often clear than bloody.

New pleuritic pain caused by heparin-induced bleeding into a site of prior infarction should not be taken to mean new embolism.

The electrocardiogram is diagnostic of pulmonary embolism in only 11% of instances.

PRINCIPLES USEFUL IN TREATMENT

Deep venous thrombosis, untreated, carries a mortality of only 1 to 2%.

Untreated pulmonary embolism carries a mortality of 20 to 25%. A patient rendered hypotensive and hypoxic by major central pulmonary embolism is in a group with a mortality rate of around 50% without treatment.

A seven- to ten-day course of heparin at therapeutic levels carries a mortality of 0.5% from intracranial, adrenal, or other hemorrhage. This complication is largely limited to older patients with hypertension or diffuse vascular disease. The heparin dosage or the risk assumed in advising venous interruption must be adjusted to these other relative risks.

Among women over 60 years of age treated with heparin in full therapeutic doses, 50 to 60% will bleed sufficiently to necessitate cessation of the drug.

Patients with migrating thrombophlebitis initiated by cancer of the pancreas, lung, or stomach have incurable tumors.

DIAGNOSIS OF DEEP VENOUS THROMBOSIS

BACKGROUND

Bed rest of five days or more.

Leg fracture or severe leg injury requiring immobilization by cast or traction.

Congestive heart failure.

New stress, e.g., major operation, myocardial infarction, pneumonia.

Pregnancy, usually late.

Prior known deep venous thrombosis.

Malignancy, especially of the pancreas, stomach, lung, or ovary.

Arterial insufficiency of the leg, reducing venous return.

Polycythemia, high hematocrit states.

Low-flow state, shock.

Age.

SYMPTOMS

Ache in the calf, worse on dependency, or ache in the medial thigh or groin. Groin ache is typical of acute iliofemoral thrombosis.

Limp, worsening with distance.

Observable swelling of the ankle, calf, or thigh.

SIGNS

Tenderness deep in the calf muscle, or over the popliteal or femoral vein.

Measurable swelling of the calf or thigh or both.

Pain in the calf muscle elicited by passive dorsiflexion of the foot on the affected side. (This sign is also positive when it occurs after a calf muscle tear or during ischemic injury to the calf musculature.)

In iliofemoral venous thrombosis, a new network of dilated intradermal veins may be visible in the affected groin.

Temperature from 99°F. to (rarely) 103°F. The latter *may* be seen in extensive iliofemoral thrombosis.

LABORATORY OR RADIOLOGIC CONFIRMATION

In a patient already subjected to five days or more of bed rest in an appropriate clinical setting who has aching discomfort, measurable swelling, and convincing tenderness, the diagnosis of deep venous thrombosis can be made with confidence on clinical grounds alone. On the other hand, leg swelling may follow any leg injury, local operation, muscle strain, thermal burns or sunburn, or cellulitis.

Impedance Plethysmography: This is not yet sufficiently reliable. Too many false-positives and too many false-negatives result from this technique.

Radioiodinated Fibrinogen Scanning: This is both cumbersome and expensive and is overly sensitive to meaningless thrombi in branch calf veins and unreliable in detecting important femoroiliac clots.

Doppler Ultrasound Recordings: Doppler ultrasound recordings of flow through major venous trunks are useful if occlusion by thrombosis is complete. However, they are unreliable when flow is maintained past a clot.

Phlebography: This is a highly accurate technique.

DIAGNOSIS OF PULMONARY EMBOLISM

BACKGROUND

The background factors are the same as those mentioned for the diagnosis of deep venous thrombosis. Pulmonary embolism is rare in people who are generally well and leading active lives. It is rare before age 30 unless several of the background factors are acting strongly together.

The presence of known deep venous thrombosis greatly strengthens the likelihood that pulmonary embolism has occurred. If lung scans are done on all patients with deep venous thrombosis who do not have chest symptoms, a significant fraction—perhaps 15 to 20%—will be found to have silent pulmonary embolism.

SYMPTOMS

Shortness of breath at rest or on minimal exertion.

Pleuritic chest pain, usually over the lower lobe of one lung (occurs on the right in 60%).

Hemoptysis (occurs in 30% of cases).

SIGNS

Respiratory rate over 20 per minute. Seen in 100% of patients with fresh pulmonary embolism.

With pleuritic chest pain there may be obvious splinting of one side of the chest.

Tachycardia.

Friction rub, often transient, denotes infarction, and is present in 30%.

LABORATORY CONFIRMATION

Arterial Blood Gas Determination: The pO_2 value when the patient is breathing room air is less than 80 mm Hg in almost every case.

Plain Chest Film: Large central emboli may produce a dilated pulmonary artery, evident oligemia of lung segments, or a dilated azygos vein. Evidences of infarction are a somewhat triangular parenchymal infiltrate based on a pleural surface, pleural fluid, or a high diaphragm.

Lung Scan: Convincing "cold defects" in areas where the chest film is clear make solid evidence for embolism. The poor perfusion of the lung bases that is the rule in congestive heart failure dictates underreading of the scan in these circumstances.

Pulmonary Arteriogram: Large central defects, cutoffs of major pulmonary arterial branches, and sharply defined segments of oligemia are caused by emboli. "Pruning" of small vessels is an equivocal finding.

TREATMENT

VENOUS THROMBOSIS

Give 5000 to 7500 units of heparin intravenously every 4 hours, the amount depending on body weight, age, and the extent of thrombosis. A major new iliofemoral venous thrombosis demands a larger dose than does a local process in a soleal vein.

Start warfarin (Coumadin) on the second day of heparin administration after obtaining a baseline prothrombin time.

Maintain the heparin until the prothrombin time has been elevated to twice the control value for three to four days. This usually means a heparin course of eight to ten days.

In venous thrombosis the Lee-White clotting time or the partial thromboplastin time is allowed to return to normal before the next heparin dose is given.

When pulmonary embolism does not accompany venous thrombosis, venous interruption procedures should not be used often but must be considered in four situations:

1. When anticoagulants are contraindicated.
2. In failures of adequate anticoagulant programs.
3. With several recurrences of deep venous thrombosis, each treated by anticoagulation.
4. In young patients with acute iliofemoral thrombosis of less than 48 hours who first present with inguinal pain.

PULMONARY EMBOLISM

About 80% of cases can be managed with heparin and warfarin. In most instances, the first dose of heparin should be 10,000 units. Subsequent doses will vary between 7500 and 10,000 units given intravenously every 4 hours, the dose depending on body weight and extent of embolism.

As with deep venous thrombosis, warfarin is added early, and heparin is discontinued by the same criteria. Warfarin therapy is maintained after hospital discharge until the patient is deemed to have returned to the original state of good health. The patients are arbitrarily blocked into treatment periods of six weeks, three months, or six months.

Patients who have been rendered hypotensive and hypoxic by major central embolism are treated initially over the first few hours of the first day by using a dose as high as 15,000 units of heparin every 4 hours intravenously. It should be recalled that elderly patients of small body build may be sensitive to heparin.

In pulmonary embolism, several clear-cut situations require that some type of venous interruption be considered:

1. When anticoagulant drugs are contraindicated.
2. When a trial of usually adequate anticoagulant therapy fails.
3. When the predisposing cause leading to embolism will continue to be present for many months or years. The best example is chronic congestive heart failure.
4. When major to massive pulmonary embolism renders the patient hypotensive and hypoxic, but he responds promptly or over hours to pressor support. In such cases, defer clipping of the inferior vena cava for 12 to 24

hours and sometimes for 36 hours until circulatory stability is assured. In the meantime, maintain high-dose intravenous heparin.

5.   When repeated episodes of pulmonary embolism require several separate periods of hospitalization.

6.   When pulmonary embolism occurs during pregnancy.

The best procedure for preventing further pulmonary embolism is compartmentalization of the inferior vena cava into four channels, each 4 mm. in diameter, by applying a serrated Teflon clip externally. No thrombus of life-threatening size can pass beyond this barrier to the lung. This operation carries a very low in-hospital mortality in patients not having chronic congestive heart failure, preexisting pulmonary insufficiency, or major sepsis.

When the patient is too ill for general anesthesia or when late-stage congestive heart failure is present, make the choice between bilateral common femoral vein ligation under local anesthesia or a Mobin-Uddin filter placed under local anesthesia down from the internal jugular vein under fluoroscopic control. Thigh swelling, implying thrombus above the common femoral level, or a phlebogram showing iliac clot dictates the use of a filter. An exception here may be the young patient seen in the first 48 hours after onset, in whom venous thrombectomy may seem worthwhile.

Common femoral vein ligation carries a 10% incidence of further embolism in unselected patients without heart disease and a 20% incidence of further embolism in similar patients with congestive heart failure. If preoperative phlebograms show no clots in the common femoral or iliac veins, these recurrence rates, while unreported, doubtless would be much lower.

CLIP COMPARTMENTALIZATION OF THE INFERIOR VENA CAVA

OBJECTIVES

To prevent both short- and long-term pulmonary embolism.
   To eliminate the need for anticoagulant drugs.

INDICATIONS

These have been outlined above.

CONTRAINDICATIONS

Major sepsis or severe chronic congestive heart failure or hypoxic lung disease antedating embolism.
   Inability of the patient to tolerate general anesthesia.

PLANNING AND PREPARATION

After major pulmonary embolism, the operation should be deferred and heparin therapy continued until normal blood pressure can be maintained without pressor support. This may require from 12 to 36 hours.

Stop heparin 4 hours before operation.

Two operative approaches to the inferior vena cava may be used. The first is upper abdominal and transperitoneal through a right subcostal incision similar to that used for cholecystectomy (Fig. 21-1). The advantage of this approach is that the clip is placed just below the well-identified renal veins, so that high-flow venous blood sweeps across the newly created venous channels to prevent thrombus formation above the clip. This operation takes longer and results in somewhat more postoperative discomfort and interference with pulmonary and intestinal function than does the extraperitoneal flank approach.

The extraperitoneal flank approach is exactly like that described in Chapter 16 for lumbar sympathectomy (Figs. 16-2, 16-3, and 16-4). In this operation, be certain to distinguish the vena cava from the right common iliac vein by identifying two sets of lumbar veins. Rule out a double vena cava (about 1% incidence), primarily by estimation of appropriate size and rarely by dissection beyond the aorta under the small bowel mesentery. Equally rare patients will have a left-sided vena cava that can be reached from the right extraperitoneal approach by extending the incision through all layers to the midline.

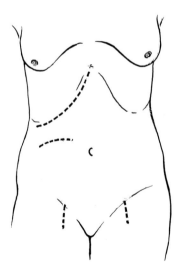

Figure 21-1. Incisions.

OPERATION

Position: Supine.

Incision and Exposure: Right subcostal from the midline to the anterior axillary line (Fig. 21-1).

After opening the peritoneum, pack off the transverse colon downward and retract in this direction with a deep Deaver retractor. Place a second gauze pad over the liver and gallbladder and arrange traction to hold these structures upward and laterally. Place a third gauze pad on the pylorus and the gastrohepatic ligament, and retract these structures upward and to the patient's left.

In the center of the resultant triangle lies the curve of the duodenum. This is a deep exposure, and accurate placement of the gauze pads and retractors is important.

Open the retroperitoneum just medial to the right kidney and just lateral to the duodenum. Extend this incision upward to the common bile duct superiorly and downward around much of the third portion of the duodenum inferiorly. Elevate the retroperitoneum in this plane laterally to the kidney, downward under the mesocolon, and medially under the duodenum to the head of the pancreas. Pick up these retroperitoneal cut edges in long stay sutures placed every 3 to 4 cm., catch the ends in Kelly clamps, and deploy these traction sutures around the field (Fig. 21-2).

Place the three retractors under the resulting retroperitoneal flaps, the medial one under the reflected duodenum.

Pick up and open the filmy areolar tissue at the junction of the right renal vein and the vena cava. Clear the anterior wall of the vena cava downward for 7 to 8 cm., staying in the plane immediately above the adventitia.

Dissection: Pick up a large bite of the anterior wall of the vena cava in a smooth forceps; clean off the fatty and filmy, weblike tissue on both sides until the confluence of two sets of lumbar veins is clearly exposed (Fig. 21-3) both laterally and medially. It may be necessary to ligate one pair of lumbar veins just below the renal vein. Pass ligatures around these fragile veins. Leave 6-mm. venous stumps.

Now pick up the entire vena cava momentarily between these lumbar veins in a smooth forceps and pass a braided silk tie in a curved vascular clamp directly beneath the tips of the forceps. This will eliminate the common hazard of injuring one of the lumbar veins.

Tie the vena cava down to a caliber of 1 cm. with an overhand throw of this temporary tie and place a hemostat on the free end of this ligature (Fig. 21-4). This partial ligature creates an open tunnel beneath the cava through

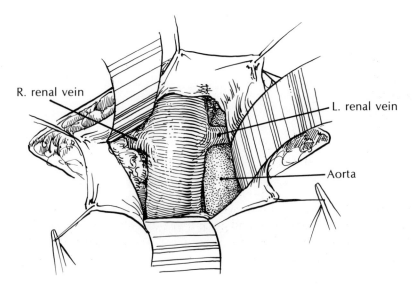

Figure 21-2.   Exposure of inferior vena cava.

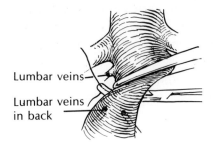

Figure 21-3.   Underpassing the vena cava.

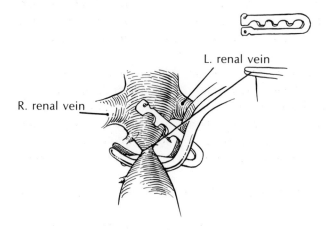

Figure 21-4.   Application of clip.

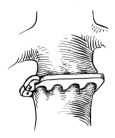

Figure 21-5.   Clip in situ.

which one arm of the serrated clip is easily passed laterally from the midline. Open the clip to about 100 degrees and grasp it in a vascular C-clamp, so that the lower arm of the clip lies within the tips of the clamp and the jaws of the clip are held firmly open by the compression of the curve of the C-clamp (Fig. 21-4).

Pass the tip of the C-clamp through the tunnel behind the vena cava, seize the anterior arm of the clip in a long clamp, and withdraw the C-clamp.

Pass a silk suture through both holes in the clip and tie it down. Place a second tie around the notches in the clip, using a surgeon's knot, and firmly tie this down. Cut out the temporary ligature of braided silk, thus allowing the vena cava to fill out within the confines of the clip (Fig. 21-5). Adjust the clip so that its long axis lies in the coronal plane. It is unnecessary to close the retroperitoneum over the clip unless cholecystectomy or some gastrointestinal procedure is to be added.

POSTOPERATIVE MANAGEMENT

Elevate the foot of the bed so that the patient's feet are higher than his heart for most of the time. Apply firm elastic stockings or bandages from the base of the toes to below the knees. Use them above the knee only if thigh swelling appears or increases.

Monitor hourly urine volumes, central venous pressure, and systemic blood pressure for the first two to three postoperative days to detect the possibility of massive pooling of blood and plasma below the clip in case of sudden closure by further embolism. If oliguria or hypotension with a falling central venous pressure should occur, give 1000 ml. of plasma rapidly intravenously, followed by another 1000 ml slowly until circulating blood volume has been restored.

Measure and record on the chart the daily maximum calf circumferences of both legs.

It is not uncommon for the clip to close between the tenth and twentieth postoperative day. This event is little reflected in blood volume shifts but presents as an iliofemoral thrombophlebitis in the "good" leg. Bed rest and marked leg elevation are more important here than is anticoagulation.

Ambulation is governed by the basic disease and the amount of leg swelling. Several short walks each day, gradually increasing in number, are ideal.

Long sitting is discouraged, and every half hour of sitting should be paid for by at least 1 hour of recumbency with the legs elevated.

Avoid postoperative anticoagulants if at all possible. Exceptions include patients with prosthetic aortic valves or recent arterial embolism. If heparin is needed for the first two or three postoperative days, again monitor the hourly urine volumes, systemic arterial pressure, and central venous pressure. Check the hematocrit frequently.

BILATERAL COMMON FEMORAL VEIN LIGATION

OBJECTIVES

To prevent pulmonary embolism.

INDICATIONS

Outlined on page 194.

CONTRAINDICATIONS

Thigh swelling.
    Severe arterial insufficiency. Major leg swelling can result in tissue necrosis.

OPERATION

Position: Supine. The table is slightly inclined with the feet down.

Anesthesia: Local infiltration plus field block. The latter is effected by depositing the anesthetic agent as a barrier at the level of, and deep to, the inguinal ligament.
    Discontinue heparin 4 hours before the procedure.

Incision and Exposure: A 10-cm. incision is made directly over the pulsating common femoral artery, with the upper end just below the inguinal ligament (Fig. 21-1; the right side is depicted).

Reflect any femoral lymph nodes medially. Try not to incise lymph nodes, since they can harbor microorganisms and incision can cause lymph leaks.

If the saphenous vein is encountered, keep the line of incision between it and the common femoral artery.

Open the deep fascia just medial to the artery. Instill additional local anesthetic agent into the femoral sheath at its upper exposure to eliminate any pain from retracting the vessels or clamping small branches.

Place one or two self-retaining retractors to hold the tissues surrounding the saphenous vein and medial leaf of the deep fascia medially and the deep fascia just superficial to the artery laterally.

Dissection: Do not dissect the artery itself. With the inguinal ligament or the saphenofemoral junction barely exposed, open the femoral sheath just medial and posterior to the artery. Enlarge the opening with the tip of a right-angled clamp and identify the common femoral vein. Clear the areolar tissue from the adventitia. Dissect the vein in this plane gently, avoiding injury to its thin-walled branches. Identify the two or three large circumflex femoral veins that pass medially, laterally, or posteriorly almost at right angles to the common femoral trunk.

Selecting Exact Level of Ligation: Work downward to identify positively the deep femoral vein takeoff, which lies almost behind the prominent valve in the superficial femoral vein (Fig. 21-6A). The deep femoral vein can be differentiated with certainty from a circumflex branch because its course diverges only slightly from the axis of the common femoral and superficial femoral veins and follows the course of the deep femoral artery, which is palpable. Ligate the common femoral vein with two silk ligatures at a level clearly above the deep femoral vein and immediately below a collateral branch so that no pouch or cul-de-sac with stagnant flow will be left (Fig. 21-6B). Be sure to leave at least one deep collateral branch above. The saphenous vein alone rarely suffices to prevent postoperative edema.

When the femoral vein is first isolated, palpate it carefully for inlying clot. Old clot will render the vein stiff and solid. Fresh clot will impart a subtle, sludgelike feel, easily overlooked unless carefully sought.

If clot is found, its upward extent and degree of adherence must be determined. Make a transverse venotomy through the anterior half of the common femoral vein. If the clot is black, rubbery, firm, stuck to the intima, and extends above the inguinal ligament, suture the venotomy and proceed to the other side.

If the clot is reddish, soft, and loose, extract it gently, looking for a smooth, rounded tip superiorly and free flow down from above. Doubly ligate the vein as before, preferably above any point of clot adherence but still below a large circumflex branch.

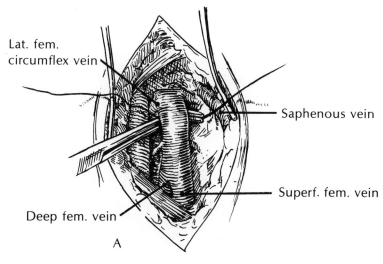
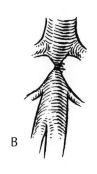

Figure 21-6.   Common femoral vein ligation. (*A*) Dissection completed. (*B*) Double ligation just below circumflex branches.

Never ligate above the saphenous vein entry and avoid ligation above all circumflex branches. Massive leg swelling requiring thrombectomy can result.

Close the deep fascia with running chromic catgut, taking pains not to pick up the saphenous or femoral cutaneous nerves.

POSTOPERATIVE MANAGEMENT

Some swelling may be expected. Elevate the foot of the bed, and apply elastic stockings.

If the iliac veins are known to be clear and no clots are encountered, omit postoperative anticoagulation. If no ligation can be done above all the thrombus, maintain anticoagulation.

Ambulation is programmed as for the caval interruption procedures.

If a lymphocele develops in the incision, leave it alone. If an open lymph leak occurs, plan for simple, bulky dressings. It will close in two to six weeks.

Index